Color Me Slim

A Path to Wellness with Vibrant Foods and Therapeutic-Grade Essential Oils

Rita M. Anderson, DCh

1st Edition: August, 2010

Edited by: Paige A. Lehmann

Cover and book design by: Matthew J. Anderson

International Standard Book Number: 978-0-9845755-0-3

Anderson, Rita M.

1. Whole Foods Diet.   2. Weight Loss
3. Essential Oils   4. Alternative Health

Important Notice

The information provided herein reflects the personal research and experiences of the author, and is for educational purposes only. It is not intended as a diagnosis, treatment or prescription for any disease or mental illness. The author, publisher and distributors accept no responsibility for such use. If you have questions as to the appropriateness of the information about your own health or may be suffering from any disease, illness or injury consult with a qualified healthcare professional.

The names of the essential oils listed are trademarked by Young Living Essential Oils, Lehi, Utah. Mention of Young Living Essential Oils does not imply endorsement by Young Living Essential Oils. All content except for cited portions is the work of a Young Living Independent Distributor, ID Number 1159, who may receive monetary compensation and/or commissions as a result of orders for products mentioned herein. The author does not have a working relationship with any company of brand named products mentioned other than Young Living Essential Oils.

Note that any statements in this book that relate to nutrition and effects of foods and nutritional supplements to health have not been evaluated by the Food and Drug Administration, and modern scientific research has not yet validated any historical claims made from empirical knowledge.

In Gratitude

These few words are meant to convey a depth and richness I feel as I acknowledge my many Teachers in my life's quest to gain knowledge and wisdom, and loved ones from whom I have received so much support. I am grateful for each of you. I wish to thank all authors whose written works have influenced my life, with special thanks to my friends and family who have inscribed their gracious words and generous ways upon my heart. Most especially thanks to my husband, Walt, who is known for living his life before all as an open book, willing to be read as a Godly, loving soul. To our children Sandra, Matthew and Peter Mark, your sweet spirits and bright, upbeat attitudes bless and inspire me. This book is dedicated to you and your families.

Thank you does not seem adequate to say to all our special associates in Young Living Essential Oils as you give of yourselves to bless and serve others. We appreciate each of you! Also, we hold Dr. Gary Young, Mary Young and all the staff at Young Living in the highest regard. With gratitude we thank them for supporting all of us, and empowering us to achieve great things.

If any copyrighted material has been quoted inadvertently, please know that my intention is not to claim originality for the work of others. I shall gladly make proper note of any omissions in subsequent book revisions.

This work is lovingly copyrighted by the Universal Law of Reciprocation. Any portion of this book lifted and posted elsewhere must include a live link back to:

www.ColorMeSlim.com

May, 2010

My Dear Family,

It has been on my heart to write you to share some key health information that I have distilled from my studies and research over the years. I've so desired to give you the benefit of my endeavors to understand what we need to become healthy, and to remain healthy. I'm concerned you may not know how very far removed we are as a nation from what is needed to be truly well, and how our natural sensibilities and receptivity to live foods have been eroded in our consciousness. Consequently, eating excessively processed foods has become the norm, and our bodies' systems are not receiving the nutrition they need to maintain balance.

Now that our nation is facing a multitude of health problems that stem from our modern diets, I decided that if I could help you understand why this is happening, then perhaps you would also be interested in learning effective ways of maintaining your health. My plan is made of four parts: 1) it's all natural, 2) it helps to restore glandular balance, 3) its main components are vibrant whole foods and therapeutic-grade essential oils, and 4) it personalizes the information because it is my story.

Please remember as you read that I am not a medical professional, and this information is not intended to replace your licensed healthcare providers. If you are ill or injured, I urge that medical services be sought. Likewise, be sure to discuss any changes in your diet or exercise if you are presently under a doctor's care or before starting a weight reduction program.

My desire is to share with you a daily celebration for all the family to enjoy for better energy, clarity of mind and body, and shedding stored fat. It is planned with the care we would give to a special holiday feast. It is a celebration of life with beautiful, wholesome foods and mindful eating. It is a path to wellness.

Fragrant blessings,

Rita Anderson

Arvada, Colorado

Contents

Section 1

"Things do not change; we change."

~ Henry David Thoreau

THE COLOR ME SLIM SECRET

You already have all you need to get started with the Color Me Slim plan, and your heart already knows the secret. It knows what is best for you, and will communicate that to you as you seek to still your mind long enough to listen. It is from this intuitive place within that you will find agreement with what is highest and best for your well being.

Your mind has been conditioned with certain beliefs about health, and perhaps what it takes to reduce weight, especially if you've tried reducing several times. Your internal knowing can direct your thoughts rather than always having external circumstances in control of your thoughts and actions. The secret is that we become what we focus on. When we give diligent thought to a plan, and set goals while taking action to move forward, we are directing our thoughts to our desired outcome. It's a process, and it's the Law of Attraction at work in our lives.

We attract into our lives what we need to succeed by being aware and alert to the twists and turns of life that open a path before us. We can hold an image of what we'd like our goal to be and see it as if it were an accomplished fact. We can choose words and actions that are uplifting and encouraging. The secret to reducing weight starts in your inner person by releasing old beliefs and consistently entertaining thoughts that support your desired outcome.

Herein lies the beauty of therapeutic-grade essential oils. When we inhale the fragrance of pure oils, their chemistry and high frequency is carried immediately to the limbic system in the center of the brain, where olfaction (smell) effects emotions. This area of the brain is closely related to the control center, or hypothalamus. We will see later how important it is to keep these glands healthy for regulating appetite to eat and thirst urging us to drink water.

No doubt you recognize some emotional reactions you have that seem to rise with no forethought of your own. These are automatic emotional responses, and some of them are tied to limiting beliefs about food, eating and your weight. The secret is that we can bring these subconscious beliefs into our conscious awareness where we can choose to clear them. In her book, Releasing Emotional Patterns with Essential Oils, Dr. Carolyn Mein, DC, comments, "The challenge in changing emotional patterns has been to access the cellular memory and change the automatic response... Changing a limiting belief requires being conscious of it and choosing a new direction."[1] Her book explains how to apply pure essential oils to facilitate the work of emotional release.

Give your heart a chance to impress you with what is possible for you and plan a path forward. When you have an image in your mind of what you'd like to create from that better, healthier perspective, then it's time to write a plan and set some goals. Desire and imagination are not enough. It is so important to take the time and make the effort to write out what it is you wish to accomplish.

THE secret is when you direct your conscious thoughts to make realistic, practical plans that agree with what your heart knows is best for you, then you will confidently move forward and attract what you need to fulfill your goals. It is my hope that the Color Me Slim concept will be a guide that will ease your way as you travel the wellness path.

THINKING OF YOU

As you hold this book in your hand, you should know that I was thinking of you, and you inspired me to write it. You pulled it out of me from near and far. Since I've allowed my weight to come into a healthy balance, and am past the learning curve, the desire to tell you some of what I have learned has increased.

Originally, my focus was not to produce a book. My focus, my reason for finally making a concentrated effort to change, is because I enjoy family life, and I intend to continue doing so for many more decades. I found this desire for healthy longevity and to fully enjoy my family to be more compelling than just wishing to be slim. I've been able to define my greater Purpose through love and service to my family; my biological and my human family.

A background of studies in holistic health, most especially my graduate work, has equipped me with resources and tools that influence the message of this book. Beyond that time, since 1994, I have continued my studies with a focus on the arts and science of aromatic essential oils applications, and Young Living Essential Oils in particular. Also, I have been associated with some very talented healers and teachers for over three decades who recognize and promote the unity of our whole mind/body/spirit.

The coursework required for me to earn my graduate degree, Doctor of Chiropathy, focused on natural, holistic health and preventive modalities. ("Chiro" denotes "with the hands" while "pathy" means "with pathos or compassion.") I believe in healing touch and that our Being always seeks our highest and best. The body will work to that end for as long as we give it what it needs to fulfill it's mission.

We are destined for Purpose. Once we become determined to define our Purpose and take steps forward to manifestation, everything in the Universe will support us to accomplish it. Deciding to make life changes are often motivated by desire to fulfill your Purpose - diet included.

Consequently, Purpose has brought me and my long-time desire to share the subjects of this book. There are many voices speaking today about the epidemic of obesity sweeping across our country. I have concluded that Color Me Slim (CMS) and the Rapid Weight Reduction (RWR) plan are valuable additions to the discussion.

I intend to develop four main ideas that you will find woven throughout this book, like a tapestry. I will take threads from my life experiences and educational background to express these four themes:

1. My plan is a total "all natural" approach. It does not depend on pre-packaged or processed foods. You will be able to find everything you need at your local grocery store, health food store, online and from a Young Living Essential Oils independent consultant.

2. The ideas presented are to work with nature for balance. Focus is brought to weight gain as a result of imblance in the body systems, including the glandular system with special attention to the endocrine system and the hypothalamus disturbances of which weight gain is a symptom.

3. Color is an expression of light as a vibratory frequency. Live foods reflect the light to us by their color and

impart their life force or vibrancy to us as we eat them. This plan is based on filling ourselves - nourishing ourselves - with the light and vibrancy of live foods, and to color our lives with "nature's living energy" found in therapeutic-grade essential oils.

4. This is my story. After over 30 years of gradual weight gain and trying many approaches to achieving and maintaining a healthy weight, it has been applying this collection of methods that have brought me my present wellness.

MINDFUL HABITS

What does it mean to develop mindful habits? You have probably heard already that it takes an average person at least twenty-one days, just 3 weeks of repetitive action, to train the psyche and neurology to respond more automatically or "by habit." This is what I mean by having mindful habits established within so you can enjoy the freedom of automatically choosing better foods, or choosing to remember why you want to be happier, healthier and slimmer without struggling to make it be so.

These thoughts need time to become reinforced impressions. At first, you will still be under the influence of the old "automatic pilot" of habits that have developed over the years. One practical example of how this can effect your weight is by reframing the old messages that urge you to clean your plate. Is it your own voice you hear commanding, "You should clear your plate"? Or maybe it subtly comes to you from an adult authority in your past who, very possibly, was of a frugal nature. Let it go, forgive them and yourself, and move on.

Practicing forgiveness toward yourself and others is a mindful habit that encompasses every aspect of health. When I learned this would be key to my being able to maintain my weight, I began thinking of instances of my relationship to food as a child that gave to me a sense of scarcity. The truth is that there was always enough, but in my youth I did not internalize the true circumstance. Therefore, I found myself much relieved of these imbalanced memories when I began forgiving myself through soul searching and the eyes of my adult understanding.

Beliefs about body-image established in childhood can follow a person with false and sometimes unfavorable impressions into adult life. Forgiveness is the path to redeem these energies both for oneself and all those who spoke or acted with cruelty. Also emotional stress of anger, grief, guilt, anxiety, fear, etc. has a negative effect on the function of the thyroid gland which regulates the rate of our metabolism.

Geneen Roth, author of, Women, Food and God, explained to Oprah Winfrey's audience how our beliefs show up in our relationship with food. She said, "If you're eating when you're bored or simply not hungry, you're essentially using food to avoid feeling your deep, meaningful feelings. In other words, you're allowing life to get the best of you; denying there is any goodness surrounding you except for the food that is there at the moment. You're basically eating because you've given up on something - some part of yourself."[2]

Mindful habits start with how we choose to direct our thoughts. There is a wise Chinese proverb that instructs us that just because birds fly over our heads, it does not mean that we should allow them to make nests in our hair. Directing our thoughts is like that. It is actively choosing to cancel negative thoughts and refuse to entertain them. As we direct our thoughts away from negative images about ourselves, and recognize thoughts that pull our energies down, we have the opportunity to forgive ourselves and others. We must seek to do this if we wish to be free of the undercurrent that pulls on us and causes stress.

Have you ever heard the question, "What's eating you?" We call it stress, depression, bitterness, etc. These negatives don't just play with our minds, they directly effect how we eat and often what and why we eat. The words we think and speak can create states of sadness and turmoil or peace and joy, and those we speak with charged emotion, especially so.

Let us embrace life, and speak words of life to one another! If we intend to make the effort by choosing a live diet like this plan, then let us also choose to define ourselves and others with positive, uplifting energy by being mindful of how we think and speak.

COLOR ME SLIM & RAPID WEIGHT REDUCTION
Section 1: Table 1 - POSITIVE AFFIRMATIONS

Accentuating the positive images you hold, and transforming negative ones about your self or circumstances into what you hope to see manifest can be strengthened by making statements as if they were true. Stand in front of your mirror,   declare these out loud, & mean it:

- I enjoy preparing and eating healthy foods.
- I am worthy of taking care of myself.
- I am surrounded by goodness and abundance. I look for beauty around me.
  Write some positive statements and repeat them every day.

COLOR ME SLIM & RAPID WEIGHT REDUCTION
Section 1: Table 2 - DEVELOPING MINDFUL HABITS

- It takes an average person at least 3 weeks of repetitive action to train the psyche and neurology to respond more automatically or by habit. Think about what it is you hope to accomplish, be clear in your mind, and allow this image to motivate you every day.

- Focus on how much you love others rather than how much you think others love you.

- Practicing forgiveness toward yourself and others is a mindful habit that encompasses every aspect of health.

- Being grateful is a mindful habit.

WORDS & ESSENTIAL OILS TO UPLIFT & INSPIRE

The following exercise is meant to elicit feelings that may arise as you look in a mirror and speak each positive word outloud to yourself. Experience each word. Write down the words that cause any measure of distress, hesitation or no response at all. You'll revisit them later.

Words that foster healthy energies are words of blessing, hope and inspiration, such as: Abundance, Adventure, Balance, Beauty, Believe, Charity, Clarity, Communication, Compassion, Consecration, Courage, Creativity, Dedication, Delight, Encourage, Endurance, Energy, Enthusiasm, Faith, Faithfulness, Favor, Flexibility, Forgiveness, Gladness, Gratitude, Happiness, Harmony, Health, Healing, Honesty, Hope, Inspiration, Integrity, Joy, Patience, Peace, Play, Power, Prosperity, Purpose, Release, Strength, Tenderness, Thanksgiving, Truth, Understanding, Vision, and Zest for Life.

Feelings are "energy in motion" otherwise known as e-motions. The fragrances and chemical compositions of therapeutic-grade essential oils reach the central brain, limbic or amygdala, by way of the olfactory pathways of the nose. This neuron activity leads directly to the brain centers that are known to be responsible for holding memories of emotion, especially trauma.[3] The properties of pure essential oils can facilitate release of the stored memory.

Releasing stored memory of trauma is just one way therapeutic-grade essential oils help us on our path to wellness, but it leads to greater freedom in managing our weight and our lives. Look for other benefits scattered throughout the book in the Section about body systems, in boxes, and the Section about Young Living Essential Oils.

WE MUST KNOW WHY

Developing new habits takes time and effort, and we must know why we choose to do so.

If I bumped into a friend I had not seen in some time and she noticed that I am now looking noticeably better and somewhat slimmer than when we last met, do you think she would ask me why I changed my diet? I'm fairly sure she would first want to know what I did to "lose" the weight. Was it easy? Was it restrictive? Did essential oils help? Did I go to some exotic health ranch or work with a special coach or personal trainer? She also sees the difference in my skin tone and complexion. "WHAT did you do?!" she asks.

It would not even occur to her to ask me WHY. Doesn't just about everybody want to be healthy, and especially to shed some pounds to feel better, look better? Yet to remain motivated we must intimately know WHY we wish to do this. We must discover our deeply motivating WHY we want to change.

So let me be the first to ask you, "WHY do you want to change your diet?" I know you want to change your diet because you are about to read my story to learn HOW I managed to slim down, and WHAT I did to look and feel so much better.

We look in the mirror and wish the reflection were thinner. Someone takes our picture and we wonder how and when did that happen? Well, guess what? Life happens, and we know deep down why "this" or "that" have become our excuses.

When you hear that I have eliminated sugars, bad fats and processed foods from my diet, you nod your head and agree that that sounds like a sensible thing to do, but is it a realistic way of life for you? That depends. Search your soul to ask yourself WHY you want to be healthier and slimmer.

When you thought about why you want to be slimmer/healthier/happier, were any of the reasons greater/larger/more important than your personal excuses? Honestly, have you noticed how self-talk habits, like making excuses, hinders your determination to make difficult decisions, especially in matters of change? True change will be elusive until your why is settled. Pause to look within to find your true desire to move forward in this area of your life and find your compelling why. You must feel fully persuaded by the reasons you'd like to be slimmer/healthier/happier. Just wishing it to happen will not give you the fortitude to stay the course.

Perhaps your answer to why seems obvious, and is clearly why you are reading this book: You're hoping that, before it joins all the other self-help and diet books in your library, you will glean a useful nugget or two. Maybe you picked it up because the words "essential oils" are included in the subtitle, and you are curious how they might work for slimming. As you follow on to know more about aromatic essences, you will realize how intimately they work with our senses, which in turn affect choices we make.

Changing the way we think about food can be twice the challenge because all of our senses must be retrained. The CMS plan addresses our needs for sensory satisfaction. I like to think that "nature knows" how to conduct matters for our natural bodies, and we can retrain our senses to notice, appreciate and prefer the beauty and fragrances of whole foods. Think about it this way:

✓ Taste - We were meant to eat live, colorful fruits, vegetables, nuts, seeds and lean proteins. Give nature a chance and the taste buds will respond favorably. with sweet, sour, salty, bitter, spicy, and other flavors.

✓ Smell - The sense of smell is very closely related to how we think our food will taste. "Mouthwatering goodness" starts with food fragrance that gets our digestive juices flowing. Not only do fresh, whole foods carry their own signature fragrances, using aromatherapy essential oils can help to curb appetite and relieve stress for better body systems' function.

✓ Sight - Beautiful and pleasing to the eye, we are naturally attracted to vibrantly colored foods so that we will be drawn to eat them and satisfy our need to nourish ourselves.

✓ Touch - The many textures and shapes of whole foods give us intimate clues about their growing patterns and their energy. Lovingly prepared meals "touch" our souls.

✓ Hearing - Crunches, slurps and yummy sighs give sensual cues that bring satisfaction to the chef, but are we listening to our bodies' responses to the foods we eat? What are they saying to us? What cues will we learn to feel and hear by being mindful of our food choices?

✓ Intuition - Consistently eating live foods may heighten our intuition about the food choices that are best for us and help restore our innate sense about food as the foundation of our well being.

Section 2

"Every human has four endowments -
self awareness, conscience, independent
will and creative imagination. These
give us the ultimate human freedom...

The power to choose, to respond, to
change."

~ Dr. Stephen R. Covey

THE CHOICE IS OURS

Presently, our country is on the verge of huge shifts and change in the way healthcare and sick care are administered. One thing is certain: an important change that we need to make is how we, as individuals, take responsibility for our own well-being. There are choices available to us that can be found outside of sick-care, where true healthcare promotes education to empower us to make wise choices, especially what we choose to eat.

In this book I celebrate the beauty and power of nature's live, whole, unadulterated foods, herbs and therapeutic-grade essential oils as my best choices for restoring and maintaining my health - including my weight. It is my story, but reflects the guidance of wise ones who have labored in the "back to nature" field that has fueled Complimentary Alternative Health in our country. The subject could be vast in scope, but I hope my distillation will pique your interest enough for you to direct your own discovery and growing confidence in making natural health choices. Remember, these are our bodies, and we can direct what goes in and on them. The choice is ours to make.

Research leaves no doubt that diet is related to killer disease conditions, and carrying extra stored fat is directly related to the deadliest three: heart disease, cancer and diabetes.[4] However, we do not have to be victims. If we change the way we think about the quality of what we eat, and adopt some new habits, we can remain healthy. Fortunately quality, colorful foods are abundantly available for most Americans.

My hope is that you understand how changing your diet and managing your weight tends to alleviate many symptoms of illness with a higher probability that you will remain disease-free, which equates to fewer visits to the doctor's office. If this is your goal, it means you must become informed and have practical experience in exercising your right to health freedoms by learning what is available to you that contributes to high-level wellness, and what may be robbing your chances of remaining disease-free. These days you will be in good company because Americans are trending toward awareness and demanding better choices. However, we cannot choose wisely if we are not aware of the choices we have.

The US Department of Health and Human Services, Centers for Disease Control and Prevention, National Center for Health Statistics, Division of Data Services, Hyattsville, MD, has been collecting data that reveals how Americans are choosing personal health care. Their statistics show that by 2007, 38% of the American population aged 18 and older were using so-called "unconventional medicine" (amounting to tens of billions of dollars, most of which was out of pocket) as some form of alternative medicine.[5] Furthermore, the World Health Organization (WHO) has chosen Traditional Chinese Medicine for "worldwide propagation to meet the health care needs of the twenty-first century."[6]

Traditional Chinese Medicine is a prime example of how 5,000 year-old precepts that depend on working with the natural flows of human systems, instead of against them, promote the value of using natural herbs and foods. These modalities work with the basic laws of nature to facilitate balance; in contrast, but not necessarily in opposition to, modern Western medicine. The former gives us choices to learn about prevention and how to remain well for longevity, and the latter works for us in disease and for emergency care when we are ill or injured. If we can adapt many of the wise principles that have been handed down and preserved for us through the ages, then we will experience benefit for our lives and be able to pass our knowledge on to the next generation.

The choices are many. Even what I am about to present to you could be overwhelming if you tackled all of it at once. When choosing to develop new habits, start with only two or three things you'd like to change. Likewise, when you see the body system lists and all the Young Living products that support those systems, realize that you will only be choosing, to begin with, two or three. You set your pace, but I suggest you start by *adding* some foods you know to be healthier before you start eliminating foods. Adding protein snacks will be helpful when you begin cutting back or cutting out the sweets.

YOUNG LIVING ESSENTIAL OILS

Section 2: Table 1 - PRODUCE WASH

Make your own produce wash to remove residue of agricultural waxes & sprays from fruits & vegetables:

- Dilute *Thieves Household Cleaner* 1 cap to 1 gallon of water & add 2 drops of *Lemon* essential oil to use as soak for fruits & vegetables, rinse well & spin or drain dry.

- Dilute *Thieves Household Cleaner* to make a spray to keep handy at the sink to spray & cleanse individual items. Rinse well.

BACK TO BASICS

I am healthier today than I was in my forties because I've learned some basic rules or Laws of Nature that I now prefer to use to maintain my health. These laws are more subtle and gradual in effect than the natural Law of Gravity, but are just as able to pull us down to earth if ignored. Years of study and observation, working as a Certified Wellness Consultant, and my personal trials and errors to address my own health and weight concerns convince me of this truth.

When there is disharmony in our minds and bodies, I believe we may be ignoring some spiritual and natural laws that would otherwise keep us stable and in homeostasis. I have some ideas about how to reorient our internal processes to work with the natural flow we're designed to have. These are not ideas of the latest fad diet or suggestions to move to the woods, raise a few chickens, and eat off the land. What I am about to share with you is a compilation of very sound advice that I have been able to experience first hand. Of course, it is not exhaustive, and I urge you to direct your personal research and add to the benefits of this eating plan that I developed from my own study and experience. I am a detail oriented person so I give many specifics, but the choice is yours to apply the information as much or as little as you wish. I, of course, feel obliged to share as much detail as I am able.

It is being offered in hopes that it will quiet the biochemical and energetic confusion of chaotic messages that may be a result of our modern lifestyle. Our bodies are designed for live, natural foods, not processed synthetics. As I said earlier, I am not a licensed professional, so if you decide to follow my plan you must make it your own. Play with it to learn healthy choices that work best for you. Repeatedly choosing them will create healthy new habits.

Again, the operative words in the previous paragraph set the theme for this book: choose and choices. We can and must mindfully choose what we are eating to give ourselves and our little ones the best chance at true health. The good news is that nature's bounty of colorful foods provides many great choices to give us the nourishment we need, and as a bonus, help us find the weight that is best for us. But, as I mentioned, our health freedoms depend on our educating ourselves and mindfully deciding to exercise our informed choices.

You will find some tools for tracking your progress and helping you establish some ideas of "before" and "after" values to learn how effective your choices have been. There is a simple self-awareness Body Systems Mini Survey included in Section 8 as a starting place to help you recognize body systems that may prefer specific or extra nutritional attention with foods and supplements. Read more about body systems and the foods that support them as well as the Body Systems Survey Results Sheet with a key to Young Living supplements and essential oils in Section 8. These guides are merely to help you get started with some simple self-awareness exercises.

There is also a suggested Daily Journal Worksheet provided for convenience when you're just getting started, but feel free to develop your own. The point is to realize that keeping track of what you are eating and how that food makes you feel is very important to your success. Plan to track what you eat and how you feel daily for at least 3 months.

WHY WEIGHT?

If we were born in another time and place, being pleasantly plump could be a sign of affluence. "Meat on the bones" once justified a man's pride by the obvious fact that he was able to provide abundant table-fare for his family. This is still true in some cultures, but being even pleasantly plump in most of American society would not be considered a compliment because of related health risks.

The contrast is striking because it demonstrates how different cultures think about food and the value placed on procuring it. America has made wonderful progress in the areas of agriculture and making sure that plenty abounds for most of us. However, in the process, some less tangible intuitional understanding has been almost lost in individual and group consciousness. Just as there are indigenous peoples who still depend on observation and understanding of nature and her gifts to survive, there was a time when our ancestors depended on having these skills. In Steve Gagne's book, Food Energetics: The Spiritual, Emotional, and Nutritional Power of What We Eat, he tells of a time when our ancestors, "...knew our food as the foundation of our blood, bones and nervous system; it was the catalyst of our thinking and way of living."[7]

We now rely mostly on the technology of machines and chemistry for food creation and distribution. Most of the rest of the world does not have the amount of food available to them - or as quickly available at some drive-through - as Americans and those in other countries who are becoming accustomed to eating our Western diet. Consequently, statistical data are proving that the American populace has been getting heavier each passing decade.[8]

The reasons are compound, and have had the drastic effect of creating chemical chaos, overburdening our bodies' systems and disturbing internal messages such as those produced by the hypothalamus and other glands. For example, researchers now know that a little hypothalamus protein called Neuropeptide Y (NPY) is an important contributor to our weight gain if its messages to stop eating are not recognized by our satiety center. Consequently, we continue to eat causing us to add to our stores of fat.

Traditionally weight gain has been thought to be a case of simple cause and effect: eat more calories than used equals fat storage and weight gain. When one consumes a greater amount of food energy (fuel measured as calories) than the amount utilized in one's daily activities, the body stores the excess energy in the form of fat. When this continues consistently over time, the effect is that the stores of fat increase. This seemingly simple equation is actually not so simple when we consider the many facets of our whole person, we find that the stressors of modern life (both internal and external) are influencing our endocrine system and, consequently, our weight. Since all of us experience stress these days from many sources (some of us handle it better than others), stress may be a key reason why our national statistics trend heavier. Lack of quality sleep is another.

Though I am a lay person relating some personal research, I have come to believe that the prime cause underlying most of the reasons why we gain weight probably has to do with the function of our glands, especially the master glands such as the pituitary and hypothalamus. The hypothalamus structure in the head is involved with orchestrating the release of hormones whose cascading effects influence blood sugar, metabolic rate, and adrenal-corticoid reactions to stress which is reflected in actions of the Autonomic Nervous System. It directs the release of chemical messengers called neurotransmitters for overall body systems to work in harmony.

Stress is a proven cause of overproduction of the neurotransmitter peptide NPY (mentioned above) resulting in appetite increase and fat storage. *Science News Digest for Physicians and Scientists* states in "Neuropeptide Y and Body Weight" that, "The main effect is increased food intake and decreased physical activity. NPY is secreted by the hypothalamus and, in addition to increasing food intake, it increases the proportion of energy stored as fat..."[9]

Any one item in the list below could impact the master glands and, with repetition, cause impaired function. Decide if you relate to or recognize any of the following causes that contribute to weight gain:

+ Lack of physical exercise. When we don't use the fuel we consume, body efficiency converts the food fuel to fat and stores it in case we need it "someday."

+ Psychological reasons, beliefs, or subconscious self-images that we have adapted about our relationships to food and eating.

+ A sense of lack, guilt, or being unforgiving toward the self or others, including self-loathing and the need to comfort or protect the self.

+ Emotions such as bitterness (affects the liver).

+ Hereditary patterns: blood sugar sensitivities.

- Carbohydrate intolerance: lack of enzymes needed to complete digestion of sugars and starches.

- Digestive insufficiency: low stomach acid causing incomplete breakdown of proteins that putrefy and create toxins that get stored in fat.

- Hormone imbalances: pituitary and thyroid output, adrenal exhaustion, excess estrogen, insufficient testosterone (for men) or progesterone (for women), hypothalamus function impairment.

- Food industry practices of hydrogenation, additives like MSG, food dyes, artificial sweeteners, etc.

- Allergies to certain foods, chemicals and environmental toxins that some individuals can't tolerate or metabolize, causing the immune system to become over active or exhausted.

- Pollutants and toxins in our cleaning supplies, cosmetics, skin creams, air, and water that kidneys and liver must attempt to filter.

- Prescription drugs and over-the-counter drugs affect some people with weight gain. (If this includes you, consult with your doctor.)

- Fast foods, processed foods, and more recently the growing inclusion of Genetically Modified Organisms (GMO) in foods such as corn, canola and soybeans.

- A really big reason for all people, but especially for the nation's children is the over-consumption of nutritionally depleted or empty-calorie, simple-sugar carbohydrates. (Most especially high fructose corn syrup known as HFCS.)

Further evidence relating to possible imbalance in endocrine system output is that it has been established that there are three events in the lives of women when they are most susceptible to gaining weight[10]:

1. At puberty when menses start
2. After giving birth
3. After menopause

If you are able to relate to any of the reasons cited, then know that you can slow the advance of internal chaos and affect change in the trend toward being overweight or obese. I had 30 years of gradual weight gain with many unsuccessful attempts at reducing. I believe I have been able to maintain my goal size at a healthy weight because I am aware of needs associated with my body systems, how stress and lack of sleep effect my endocrine system, and what diet plus supplements my body prefers to maintain balance.

My plan is to eat a variety of foods chosen mostly by color categories and to include extra nutritional support for body systems while limiting and eliminating known substances that are detrimental to health. The plan also calls for active participation in stress awareness and release activities. It is designed to very quickly get the body receiving what it needs to restore and rebuild health.

Along the way, it is my hope that many others will re-establish that lost cultural intuition about our food that our ancestors understood as the foundation of our blood, bones and nervous system, and the catalyst of our thinking and way of living.

COLOR ME SLIM

Section 2: Table 2 - CMS BASICS

- Balanced meals of vibrantly colored carbohydrates, fats & complete protein.
- Daily Journal for tracking.
- Assess for awareness of balance and to identify priority body systems.
- Hydrate & flush toxins with plenty of pure water.
- Practice stress release for needed rest, digestion and appetite control.
- Includes using therapeutic-grade essential oils & oil-enhanced supplements.

COLOR ME SLIM

Section 2: Table 3 - THE FOOD CATEGORIES

A complete CMS cleansing and balancing diet will include:

- **COMPLETE PROTEIN**
- **GREEN VEGETABLES**
- **ROOT VEGETABLES**
- **GREEN LEAFY VEGETABLES**
- **RED, ORANGE & PURPLE VEGETABLES**
- **YELLOW, PALE GREEN, & WHITE VEGETABLES**
- **BEANS, SEEDS, GRAINS & NUTS**
- **FATS & OILS**
- **FRUITS & MELONS**
- **HERBS & CONDIMENTS**
- **WATER, HERBAL TEAS & BEVERAGES**

Are you able to name how many different vegetables and fruits you have consumed in the last month? Do you have salads made of the same boring three or four items? If so, are you ready to embark on a bit of kitchen and culinary adventure? Again, not to worry. It will perfectly agree with the CDC diet guidelines.[11] If you are like most Americans, you have probably been eating certain foods for reasons other than nutritional value, and there is a good chance your diet would not be considered a cleansing and building diet. You have probably also been eating a limited number of food types.

We start with a basic plan that features food variety to help build the body's defenses. The Color Me Slim plan provides for maximum nutrition and helps to minimize allergies because the diversity of colorful food available to us allows us to rotate our many different choices. Rotation is one way to manage or avoid the overload of allergens and toxins that cause allergies. When we eat certain foods of similar families too frequently, allergies may result. Giving your body the fibrous roughage and varied enzymes characteristic of many colorful plant foods can limit the possibilities of food sensitivities or ease food allergies.

ORGANIZING MENUS BY COLOR

Allowing color to dominate how you organize your menus is a simple way to ensure that you give your body good, balanced fuel for energy. Many red fruits and vegetables serve as blood builders along with the other nutrients they provide the body. In the same way, yellow foods can serve the body as laxatives. Also green foods, such as avocado, cucumber, broccoli, spinach, beans, parsley, etc., have the power of purifying and building the blood and rejuvenating the body as a whole.[12]

Steve Gagne' explains in his book, Energetics of Food - Encounters with Your Most Intimate Relationship, "Light is food to the photosynthetic plant kingdom. The six basic colors are the Warm to Hot colors - yellow, orange and red - and the Cool to Cold colors - green, blue and purple. Each of the warmer colors has a complementary cooler color, and vice versa. Creative cooks implement a balanced color scheme in their preparations to create appealing and satisfying meals. The most energizing meal is one that includes a mix of both warm-and-cool-colored foods."[13]

I've organized colorful warm-and-cool fruits and vegetables into a plan I call Color Me Slim or CMS. Whenever I follow CMS my health improves, and my weight stabilizes. I've learned what works, and how to simplify preparation to be able to maintain the plan even when I have a busy schedule. You will find these helpful tips scattered throughout the book.

THE COLOR ME SLIM FOOD CATEGORIES

CMS & RWR

Section 2: Table 4 - COMPLETE PROTEIN

Meats: Beef, buffalo, chicken, cold water fish, eggs, lamb, lobster, sardines, shrimp, turkey, & wild game. (Beef is not eaten two days in a row, and never twice in the same day.) Grass-fed, or free-range organic meats when possible. No deli meats, nitrates or nitrites. No fried meats. No flour breadings or coatings.

Cheese: Cottage cheese (1% fat or non-fat), Greek yogurt (non-fat), hard cheeses, jack or mozzarella cheese (reduced fat), Ricotta cheese, New Zeland whey

Protein Powders: Rice protein, whey protein, soy protein (limit, no GMO). Use New Zeland whey. Limit or eliminate soy.

Eggs: Fresh, from true "cage-free" or "free-run" chickens or ducks.

Milk: Almond milk, coconut milk, cow milk (organic non-fat or 1%), goat milk, rice milk, hemp milk. (NO soy milk unless you can be sure it is GMO-free source -- then limit use.)

CMS & RWR

Section 2: Table 5 - YELLOW, PALE YELLOW, PALE GREEN, & WHITE VEGGIES

Avocado, Bamboo Shoots, Bean Sprouts, Bok Choy, Celery, Cauliflower, Corn (fresh), Fennel, Garlic, Green Onions, Jicama, Mushrooms, Onions, Scallions, Sprouts, Summer Squash, Turnip, Yellow Wax Beans, Yellow Tomato, Zucchini

CMS & RWR

Section 2: Table 6 - RED, ORANGE, & DARK PURPLE VEGGIES

Beets, Carrots, Eggplant, Pumpkin, Purple Cabbage, Red Peppers, Rutabaga, Sweet Potato, Tomato, Yams

CMS & RWR

Section 2: Table 7 - GREEN LEAFY VEGGIES

Arugula, Beet Greens, Bok Choy, Cabbage, Chard, Chicory Greens, Cilantro, Collards, Kale, Mustard Greens, Parsley, Spinach, Watercress

CMS & RWR

Section 2: Table 8 - GREEN VEGGIES

Artichoke, Asparagus, Bell Peppers, Broccoli, Celery, Green Chilies, Cucumber, Green Beans, Leaf Lettuces, Leeks, Okra, Romain Lettuce, Sprouts (alfalfa, chia, flax, mung, sunflower)

As you can see, different categories of fresh, whole foods are represented according to their color groups. Both warm-colored and cool-colored foods are found in each group. Refer to these categories to build shopping lists and when converting favorite family recipes. Choose at least one item from EVERY category every day. It's even better to eat several of each category every day. The more variety you choose, the greater chance of balancing your diet. By following the list of foods while shopping, you will be able to quickly determine if you have enough of each category.

If you are buying mostly fresh and raw, there won't have to be too much label reading. However, there are certain packaged items with labels that you will absolutely want to inspect closely to be certain that you are not inadvertently buying sugars, salt and some soy (and meat analogues made from soy). It's just easier to eat fresh, whole foods than having to worry about avoiding hidden ingredients.

The actual plan is fairly simple. Each day choose your breakfast, lunch, and dinner by including one or more of each food type to ensure that you have eaten a colorful variety that day. Drink a protein-rich smoothie or eat fruits and protein as snacks between meals. That's it!

It's simple, but not necessarily easy because a few of our favorite tastes and stimulants are restricted (as in gradually eliminated) going forward. However, after just a few days of eating unlimited amounts from these food lists and applying therapeutic-grade essential oils to help with releasing possible emotional attachments to sweet and stimulating foods, you'll be feeling much better and won't be craving the stimulants as much.

CMS & RWR

Section 2: Table 9 - ROOT VEGGIES

Beets, Carrots, Jicama, Kohlrabi, Parsnips, Potatoes, Radish, Rutabaga, Sweet Potatoes, Turnips, Yams, Water Chestnuts

CMS & RWR

Section 2: Table 10 - FRUITS

Apples, Apricots, *Bananas, Black Berries, Blueberries, **Cantaloupe, Cherries, *Dates, Cranberries, *Figs, Grapes, Grapefruit, Guava, Kiwi, Lime, Litchi, Mango, **Melons, Nectarine, Oranges, Papaya, Passion Fruit, Peaches, Pears, Pineapple, Pomegranate, Raspberries, *Raisins, Star Fruit, Strawberries, Tangerine, **Watermelon   *high sugar, limit   **For best digestion, eat melons alone.

CMS & RWR

Section 2: Table 11 - BEANS, PEAS, SEEDS, GRAINS & NUTS

Adzuki Beans, Black Beans, Black Eyed & Cow Peas, Fava Beans, Garbanzo Beans (Chickpeas), Kidney Beans, Lentils, Lima Beans, Pinto Beans, White Beans, *Peas,Amaranth, Brown Rice (long grain), Kamut, Oatmeal, Quinoa, Rye, Spelt, Teff, *Whole Wheat, Chia Seeds, Flaxseeds (fresh ground), Pine Nuts, Pumpkin Seeds, Sunflower Seeds, Almonds (soaked), *Brazil Nuts, *Cashews, Filberts,*Macadamia, *Peanuts, *Pecans, *Pistachios, *Walnuts, (All seeds and nuts are raw, unsalted & unroasted.) *limit

CMS is a plan designed to answer the need to get back to whole food eating without the packaged foods and fast foods that may be laced with chemicals and preservatives and possibly prepared from genetically modified food sources. You may eat and live with the CMS plan as long as you like because it is full of the variety needed for good nutrition, fiber and other health building elements. Some health advocates believe that we cannot become fully well if eating packaged and processed foods.

It can help you slim down to eat this way, but to take significant weight off, use CMS as your foundation and continue into the second half of this book, which is dedicated to Rapid Weight Reduction (RWR). Let's face it though, most people are going to begin to drop pounds just by eliminating pretzels, chips and other carbohydrates or fatty-protein snacks. We'll expect you will look for healthier options for sodas and sugars too.

Following CMS is slimming because, by doing so, you are eliminating less beneficial chemistry in exchange for the chemistry nature uses to cleanse and build strong bodies from plenty of fruits and veggies along with lean meats and fresh eggs, herbs, seeds and nuts. When you are deciding what you want to eat, there are a few things to remember that can guide you to the best choices by considering:

+ Freshness - The fresher, more colorful, the better.

+ Calorie dense - How high is the Glycemic Index or Glycemic Loading score? Lower is better.

+ Variety - Are you eating a good variety of each food category rather than always choosing the same foods, the same colors? Be adventuresome!

CMS & RWR

Section 2: Table 12 - CONDIMENTS, HERBS & SPICES

Lemon Juice, Organic Apple Cider Vinegar, Liquid Aminos, Carob Powder, Cayenne Pepper, Cinnamon, Clove, Garlic & Onion Powders, Maple Syrup (limit), Molasses (limit), Paprika, Black Pepper, Red Wine Vinegar, Unrefined Sea Salt, Sesame Gosimo, Stevia Extract, Tahini, Tamari (wheat-free), Basil, Celery Seed (not celery salt), Chives, Dill, Fennel, Garlic, Marjoram, Mint, Oregano, Sage, Parsley, Savory, Tarragon, Thyme

READ LABELS: No salt or sugar in bottled herbs & spices.

CMS: Use a limited amount of organic Agave in place of rice bran syrup, maple syrup or honey.

RWR: Use powdered stevia or *Stevia Extract*.

CMS & RWR

Section 2: Table 13 - FATS & OILS

Butter (organic!)

Coconut Oil (virgin organic)

Olive Oil (extra virgin organic),

Almond Oil

Grape Seed Oil

Macadamia Nut Oil

Walnut Oil

Almond Butter, Cashew Butter, & Peanut Butter

(Organic & limit to no more than

2 X per week.)

COLOR ME SLIM - THE CMS PLAN

CMS is a plan to help you develop good habits that may require changes in the way you think about the types and quality of your foods, but it will be a process like anything else in life. To be successful with CMS, you don't have to be a purest, eating only the freshest organic produce or just picked from your garden! Do the best you can by eating what is available at your locale, and take care to wash produce well to remove agricultural chemical residue. Being mindful about your choices should not be stressful.

Select some of each color group every day. This will create the balance you need. CMS tips to get you started:

▸ When a food item appears in two color categories, it counts for only one. Be sure to eat something from both categories that day. Example: Red radishes are a root veggie, but they are also found in the Red, Orange, and Purple category. Count them in either one of the categories for that day or that meal, but not both.

▸ The right kind of salt is important, but just a little goes a long way. To ensure your daily amount of salt, measure some unrefined sea salt into a little bowl (only 1/4 to 1/2 teaspoon). Sprinkle from this amount throughout the day to prepare your meals. Meanwhile learn to replace other sources of salt and packaged seasonings with fresh and dried herbs for flavor and antioxidants.

▸ Protein is to be eaten at each meal and with each snack for the first 3 days of the Color Me Slim plan. Eat plenty of protein foods the first 3 days of CMS to off set the stress of eliminating and cleansing starches and sugars.

▸ Vegetarians or vegans will want to be especially certain to eat a variety of fruits, vegetables, grains, seeds and nuts to ensure they get enough protein for their bodies to formulate complete protein.

▸ Choose good fats: organic extra virgin olive oil, organic butter (see Better Butter recipe), organic coconut oil, essential fatty acids - especially Omega 3 such as Young Living's *Omega Blue*, and oil-soluble supplements of A, D, and E in your complex.

▸ Beef & Tuna: Eat only two times a week, and never twice in the same day or two days in a row to avoid high fats and sodium loading while taking longer to digest.

▸ Breads: Find sprouted whole grain or flourless breads that are low in sugar, such as Ezekiel. Cut a slice in half or only use one slice for a sandwich if it is as high as 100 calories per slice. Look for smaller-sized loaves with a profile of 50 calories or less per serving.

▸ Starches: Restrict all starches to 2 daily servings. If you have the above sandwich of a 100 calorie bread slice, then that meets your starch serving for the day. One piece of 50 calorie toast with breakfast would allow another starch serving at lunch or dinner of 1/2 medium boiled potato or yam, 1/4 cup quinoa, or brown rice (only 3 times per week combined), bread, rye crackers, 1/2 a tortilla or pita. Any type of potato is least favored because it converts to sugar so quickly.

- Coffee: Drink Green tea, Yerba Mate or Wu Long herb tea instead as a good wake-me-up.

- Water: Oxygenate and flush toxins with pure, filtered, non-chlorinated water.

- Read and follow CLEANSING HABITS suggestions in Section 5 of this book.

- Understand FOOD INTOLERANCE and realize these digestive upsets can be addressed. See Rapid Weight Reduction in Section 4 of this book.

- Read and understand WHAT YOU MAY EXPERIENCE in Section 5 of this book.

You probably are eager to learn just what I mean when I say certain foods are restricted and eliminated, but start by adding colorful vegetables and lean protein for several days before consciously avoiding foods. In CMS you can definitely begin to eat according to the color variety plan and begin to eliminate some of the less desirables, but for Rapid Weight Reduction, they will all be completely avoided. You should stay with CMS basics until your bowels are regular and you are able to truly clear your palate from cravings for salts, fatty foods and sugars.

Before you read the list, know that there really are healthier replacements for each item. Become creative with natural ingredients, and soon you will not crave any of the foods like the ones listed below. However, sugar is one culprit that should be eliminated cold-turkey - which also means any foods containing any form of sugar. Here's the CMS restricted foods list:

- Sugars - Say no to candies, cakes, cookies, pies, muffins, bagels, fruity drinks, honey, maple syrup, catsup, sodas, "sugar free" and artificial sweeteners. You MUST read labels to eliminate all sugars. (You can receive adequate natural sugars from fruit snacks and a minimal amount of food starches).

- Sodium - Skip the chips, dips, crackers, pretzels, packaged foods, fast foods, most frozen foods, soy sauce. You must read labels and compare among brands.

- Caffeine - Limit then eliminate coffee, black tea, colas, sodas, foods with caramel color, chocolate. (Unless it's super, super pure chocolate - then a little is OK - that is if you can eat only a little bit and be satisfied.)

- Creamy - No ice cream, icings, cream fillings, cream cheese or soft cheeses.

- Gravies & Sauces - No flour or cornstarch thickened meat drippings, sweet and sour sauces, soy sauce.

- Unfit Fats - No canola oil, soy oil, corn oil, lard, margarine, meat grease, mayonnaise, hydrogenated oils, FRIED FOODS, processed cheeses.

- MSG - No, not, never monosodium glutamate or glutamate-containing foods.

- Salad Dressings - No bottled salad dressings made with any vegetable oils other than organic olive oil; no non fat or low-fat salad dressings if made with artificial sweeteners or other sugars.

- Dairy - No sugar sweetened yogurts, soft cheeses, full-fat pasteurized milk, chocolate milk, dark yellow cheeses, processed cheeses made from vegetable oils, powdered cheese mixes.

▸ Flours - No refined flours, especially bleached wheat flour, and cornstarch (no "white" flour bakery foods).

YOUNG LIVING ESSENTIAL OILS
Section 2: Table 14 - SUPPLEMENTS & ESSENTIAL OILS

When shopping for food, making educated choices has become a necessity if you want to remain healthy. This includes educating yourself about the supplements and essential oils you are buying. You may not always have the best choices available in food selections, but you can always opt to buy the highest quality in essential oils and supplements.

You are invited to direct your persoanl research to the Young Living line of therapeutic-grade essential oils and their supplements enhanced with these pure essential oils. You will want to learn about basic products that give nutritional support with CMS and for RWR, such as:

- Vitamins & Minerals
- Essential Fatty Acids
- Digestive Enzymes
- Calcium/Magnesium/Potassium/Zinc
- B-Complex
- Thermogenic Herbs
- Probiotics
- Cleansing Herbs
- Protein Powders
- Hormone System Support
- Antioxidant Nutrition
- Essential Oils for Stress & Emotional Release
- Essential Oils for Cleansing & Immune System Support.

SERVING SIZES AND PORTIONS

Portion size is fundamental to weight management because people gain weight when they eat more calories than they expend. A CDC article, "Do Increased Portion Sizes Affect How Much We Eat," reports on marketing trends toward larger quantity says that, "Americans are surrounded by larger portion sizes at relatively low prices. ...The cost to America's health may be higher than most people realize. ...There are short-term studies showing that controlling portion sizes helps limit calorie intake, particularly when eating high-calorie foods."[14]

Portion sizes you need will depend on your level of activity, health, etc. In the beginning, measuring and weighing food is a great way to learn how much you are serving. Once familiar with portions of meats and fish to approximate the serving sizes suggested by the Dietary Guidelines for Americans (DGA) list,[15] you will seldom feel the need to weigh food anymore, but it is a good practice when you begin watching your portion sizes.

Try the idea of eating the amount of meat that would fit in the palm of one hand as one protein serving. Two hands cupped together filled with a colorful mix of vegetables and/or salad is perfect for an individual's serving of each. (For example, my cupped hands hold about two cups of a mixed salad or 1 cup of veggies and 1 cup of a green leafy salad. This is plenty for me.) Can you imagine portions on children's plates being more age and individual appropriate if the serving sizes were measured in this simple manner by the size of their hands? Also consider that healthy snacking at certain times of the day helps with portion control at meal time for both children and adults.

Speaking of children, Dr. L. H. Epstein and his colleagues developed The Traffic Light Diet for use in their family based childhood research. Their research features colorful foods, and as its name implies, traffic light colors of red, yellow and green are three groups of food categories intended to teach children to eat nutritious "go for the green" foods, and to "red light" foods that are not healthy choices. The plan includes age related foods and portions which should be helpful information for parents and those who prepare school and school lunch programs.[16] If you are concerned about this important issue, their program may be a good resource for you to investigate.

Be mindful of the amount you are eating of the different food categories. Become aware of serving sizes and portion control. Check ingredient labels on everything from breads to peanut butter to learn the actual calorie count, fats, sugars and sodium. When you eat out, don't expect to be served proper portions. Expect to carry a box home of at least half the portion from most restaurants because menu selections these days are at least two servings.

Look for firm breads made with whole grains, and eat no more than two slices per day at about 50 calories each. Refined flour foods are usually high on the Glycemic Index so replace all refined, white flour products with whole grain ones that carry a better Glycemic Load profile and help slow the release and absorption of glucose. Limit breads, crackers, pasta, rice, potatoes and quinoa to about 60 starch calories in a meal. Again, if you have a piece of 50 calorie toast with breakfast then one-half a sandwich at lunch, you have eaten two starch servings for that day so do not eat any yams or brown rice at supper. Though we need to eat complex starches, it is easy to overdo, slowing fat reduction.

Grain-based foods such as cakes, cereals, cookies, crackers and breads are carbohydrates that are readily converted to glucose sugar. Most bakery goods are prepared with refined flours, sugars and fats of questionable sources. Refined flours are used to prepare packaged foods for longevity on store shelves.

Limit total starch calories eaten to around 100 per day, including any starch vegetables such as potatoes, yams, squash or pumpkin. Choose whole grains, breads or crackers from the list that follows:

- amaranth - ancient grain, staple of the Aztecs
- barley - bread or cereal (limit)
- buckwheat - 1/4 C hot cereal, thermogenic for winter months, (limit)
- corn - white or yellow tortillas 1/2 (limit corn products) blue corn tortillas only 1/3 or limit to 60 calories or less per serving
- kamut - an ancient wheat-type grain
- millet - bread, 40-50 calorie slice, 1/4 C cereal (limit)
- oats - organic rolled oats 1/4 to 1/2 C (Eat only occasionally if you feel the need for more variety.)
- rye - bread or crackers, adjust amount by limiting to 50 calories or less
- rice - organic long grain brown rice, 1/4 to 1/2 C as starch serving; have this type of starch only 3 X per week.
- spelt - bread 50 calories or less, may need to cut a larger slice of 100 calories to make 2 servings

- teff - high fiber and protein, nutty flavored warm cereal
- quinoa - 1/4 to 1/2 C cooked as starch serving. Eat this type of starch only 3 X per week.
- whole wheat - bread 50 calorie or less, 1 slice or cut in half, pita 1/2

Sugars and refined flour products top the list of foods to avoid for a healthy lifestyle and longevity. It takes three to seven days to flush sugar residues from the body so drinking plenty of water is very important. Again, the rules for restricted foods bear repeating for an important emphasis. They are:

- Sugar - #1 most necessary to avoid if you want to reduce weight and regain health. It can be done! candies, cakes, cookies, pies, fruit drinks, honey, maple syrup, catsup, sodas, "sugar free" and artificial sweeteners. (No more HFCS, high fructose corn syrup!)
- No pre-packaged, processed foods - full of sugars, sodium and fats
- Nix all MSG monosodium glutamate, glutamate containing foods, flavor enhancers, soy protein isolates and other excitotoxins.
- Limit sodium - No chips, dips, crackers, pretzels, salted nuts.
- Limit caffeine, then eventually eliminate - coffee, black tea, colas & sodas, caramel colored items, chocolate
- Alcohol only on special occasion - beer, wine, liquors.

- Creamy -   No ice cream, icings, cream fillings, soft cheeses.

- Gravies & Sauces - No flour or cornstarch thickened drippings of fats and sodium, high sodium soy sauce.

- Unfit Fats - No canola oil, soy oil, corn oil, lard, meat grease, mayonnaise, hydrogenated oils like shortening and margarine; or partially hydrogenated ingredients found in many nut butters, baked goods and other packaged foods, roasted nuts.

- Meats - No pork sausage, hot dogs, bacon or processed deli meats, cold cuts, canned meats, and no breading or frying.

Section 3

"You cannot solve any problem
in the same state of consciousness
in which it was created."

~ Albert Einstein

THE DAILY JOURNAL

Every exercise or weight management plan I have come across insists on keeping a journal to track progress. It is important to your success. I have prepared one that's easier to maintain than most I've seen. When you begin CMS by gradually eliminating the restricted foods, you are choosing to make your changes as rapidly or as slowly as suits you. Tracking progress will be an especially revealing habit to develop.

The Daily Journal may be used as a guide to know what to eat and what not to eat. It is positioned in this book between the basic CMS eating plan and Rapid Weight Reduction (RWR) and can be a preview to the RWR plan. Following the lists presented on the Journal will alert you to those areas you have yet to adapt when you are ready to proceed to RWR.

CMS persons pick-and-choose daily items according to the pace and personal goals they set. However, if you suspect carbohydrate intolerance and wish to modulate your diet to find your optimal level of carbohydrate intake and/ or have made the personal commitment to reduce more rapidly, you will have had the opportunity to review the Journal each day while on CMS. You will be well aware of what is to be completed each day on RWR before you commit to it. Again, informed personal choices lead to health freedom.

As you circle your responses each day, you will become more aware of the good work you are accomplishing because each item mentioned is designed to remind you of your daily goals. By contrast, you will also be more aware of any segment that is lacking attention so you can resolve to do it if you so choose.

The self-analysis or self-awareness surveys found later in this Section should be guides to get you started with more specifically directed nutrition, giving attention to priority body systems. Study which foods, herbs and essential oils have been traditionally used for the different body systems in Section 8 and incorporate them as you plan your meals and supplements considering the priority body systems that would prefer extra nutrition.

Mark your Daily Journal as you notice any differences. After a month, a retest will most likely reveal that the priority body systems have shifted.

THE DAILY JOURNAL WORKSHEET

Name_____Date_____

Stand before a mirror. If you choose to wear clothes, wear the same clothing each time you measure.

I weighed _____ this morning. Body fat was _____% Hydration was _____%.

❖ My chest measurement is _____.

Measure the chest at nipple level.

❖ My waist measurement is _____.

Bend to the side, measure waist at crease.

❖ My lower abs measurement is _____.

Measured at the widest spot or about 2" below the navel.

❖ My hips measure _____.

Hips are measured at the widest area around.

❖ My thighs measure _____ R _____ L

Mark thighs about 9" above each knee then measure around.

❖ My calves measure _____ R _____ L

Calves are measured at about mid-calf while standing.

❖ My upper arms measure _____ R _____ L

Upper arms are measured at about mid-arm.

❖ I now wear a size _____ shirt/blouse and a size _____ pants.

❖ My blood pressure is _____/_____.

Some grocery and drug stores have blood pressure stations or you can buy a small, personal unit to use.

Plan your start day to be a Thursday if you think it might be easier to handle any craving urges over the weekend. These usually pass by the third day.

Each day's Journal may be different. Review ahead to be ready for coming changes, especially when progressing into RWR. Make blank copies of the following Daily Journal pages to allow for at least 4, to as many as 12, weeks of Journals.

✓ Check or circle all that apply.

Day 1

I choose to remember anything for which I wish to forgive myself, especially food and eating related.

☐ I took starting measurements.

☐ On this first day I am grateful to have all I need to succeed to be healthy and happy.

☐ I ate a good breakfast. I am eating extra protein for 3 days to prepare my body for the transition from eating sugars, starchy carbs, sodas, unfit fats, sodium and caffeine.

☐ I ate 1 or 2 apples or 1 or 2 small grapefruit today as snacks.

☐ I cleaned out the refrigerator and freezer.

☐ I removed any tantalizing foods from shelves and pantry.

☐ I took inventory of foods, snacks and condiments I have that I can use.

☐ I started a shopping list.

☐ I ate plenty of raw vegetables today from the colorful veggie categories (green leafy), (green), (red, purple, & orange), (yellow & white) & (root veggies).

☐ I took digestive enzymes and supplements I had available.

☐ I drank 1-2-3-4-5-6-7-8-9-10 glasses of pure water with a drop of *Lemon, Peppermint* or *Grapefruit* essential oils (EOs) 1-2-3 times.

☐ I did not eat cooked vegetables, cereals, breads or flour products today.

☐ I did not eat any deli meats, canned meats or pork products.

☐ I did not eat any starchy carbs like corn, rice, beans, potatoes or pasta.

☐ I did not eat any condiments like mayonnaise, mustard, ketchup or any seasonings that contain salt or sugar.

☐ I did not drink any dairy products, fruit juices, sodas or sweet beverages, or more than 2 cups of coffee or regular black tea. I am going to drink Green tea, Yerba Mate tea and other herb teas instead of coffee.

☐ My positive affirmation for today is:

_____

_____

_____

_____

Day 2

I'm remembering to forgive myself and others who influence how I think about food and eating.

☐ I weighed _____ this morning.

☐ I ate a good breakfast. Day 2 of protein-loading to help my body for the transition from eating sugars, starchy carbs, sodas, sodium & caffeine.

☐ I developed a preliminary food plan for the next 6 days and made a shopping list.

☐ I shopped at the Farmers' Market, grocery store, and/or health food store. I read labels.

☐ I washed fruits and vegetables and prepared them for storage. Veggies are: (green leafy), (green), (red, purple, & orange), (yellow & white) & (root veggies). Fruits to have for snacks are apples, grapefruits, oranges, blueberries & strawberries.

☐ I readied some chopped veggies in separate bins or green bags for quick use.

☐ I drank herb tea, 1-2-3 cups.

☐ Today I measured out and used 1/4 to 1/2 teaspoon total of unrefined sea salt, for my day's ration of 1500 mg or less.

☐ I ate 1 or 2 apples or 1 or 2 small grapefruit today as snacks.

☐ I am protein-loading today so I ate 1-2-3-4-5-6 servings of lean protein.

☐ I included either apple cider vinegar, red wine vinegar and/or fresh lemon juice as salad dressing with each protein meal.

☐ I took digestive enzymes and supplements I had available.

☐ I did not eat cooked vegetables, cereals, breads or floury products.

☐ I did not eat any dairy products (cheese, cottage cheese) or deli meats, canned meats or pork products.

☐ I did not eat any starchy carbs like corn, beans, rice, potatoes or pasta.

☐ I did not eat any condiments like mayonnaise, mustard, ketchup or any seasonings that contain salt or sugar.

☐ I did not drink any dairy products, fruit juices, sodas or sweet beverages, or more than 2 cups of coffee or regular black tea.

☐ I made 1-2 protein shake with water for snack today.

☐ I drank 1-2-3-4-5-6-7-8-9-10 glasses of water with *Lemon, Peppermint* or *Grapefruit* essential oils in 1-2-3 glasses.

☐ I am aware to use only therapeutic-grade essential oils.

☐ On a scale of 0 to 10 my energy was ____, my mood was ____, food cravings for sweet or salty were ____ overall I felt ____.

☐ I will drink a cup of warm lemon peel tea before going to bed tonight for cleansing.

☐ I've told at least 1-2-3 persons about my 4-week commitment.

☐ I am grateful for:

_____

_____

Day 3

Today is the last day of all I can eat of protein foods and raw vegetables before I begin eating servings the size of my hands.

☐ I weighed _____ this morning.

☐ I got 6-7-8-9 hours of sleep last night.

☐ I drank a cup of warm lemon juice tea first thing upon arising this morning to help stimulate bile and clear the liver and bowels.

☐ I ate a good breakfast that included plenty of protein and some healthy fats.

☐ I took supplements: Vitamin/Mineral 1-2-3-4-5-6, Essential Fatty Acids (EFAs) 1-2-3-4, Digestive Enzymes 1-2-3-4-5-6, Ca/K/Mag 1-2-3-4, Extra B-Complex 1-2, Thermogenic Herbs 1-2-3-4-5-6, Probiotics 1-2-3, Cleansing Herbs 1-2-3-4, Other

_____

_____

☐ I drank 1-2-3-4-5-6-7-8-9-10 glasses of pure water with *Lemon, Peppermint* or *Grapefruit* essential oils in some.

☐ I ate 1-2-3-4-5 servings of lean protein today. Last day of protein-loading preparing my body to transition to my new way of eating starting tomorrow.

☐ I ate at least 1-2-3 portions of each vegetable category today; (green leafy), (green), (red, purple, & orange), (yellow & white) & (root veggies).

☐ Today I measured out and used 1/4 to 1/2 teaspoon total of unrefined sea salt, for my day's ration of 1500 mg or less.

☐ I used fresh lemon juice and apple cider vinegar in salads or on food.

☐ I ate 1 or 2 apples or 1 or 2 small grapefruit today as snacks.

☐ I drank 1-2-3 cups of herb tea today: Green tea, Yerba Mate, Wu-Long Slimming Tea, Peppermint tea, or Chamomile tea.

☐ I made 1-2 protein shake with water for snack today.

☐ Tomorrow I may eat lightly cooked vegetables, breads or flour products, but I did not eat them today.

☐ I did not eat any dairy products (cheese, cottage cheese) or deli meats, canned meats or pork products.

☐ I did not eat any starchy carbs like corn, beans, rice, potatoes or pasta.

☐ I did not eat any condiments like mayonnaise, mustard, ketchup or any seasonings that contain salt or sugar.

☐ I did not drink any dairy products, fruit juices, sodas or sweet beverages, or more than 2 cups of coffee or regular black tea.

☐ I stretched, walked, did yoga, bounced on a mini-trampoline, or moved my lymph with a massage (w/out oil), or other form of exercise today.

_____

_____

☐ I took cleansing breath today, and did some form of relaxation for stress relief: warm bath, dry skin brushing, meditation, laughed out loud, used essential oils for Aromatherapy.

☐ On a scale of 0 to 10 my energy was ____, my mood was ____, food cravings for sweet or salty were ____ overall I felt ____.

☐ I reviewed or revised my food plans for the rest of the week to make sure I have everything I need: foods, spices, and supplements.

☐ I meditated, read, got fresh-air and sunshine, hugged someone, played a game, told a joke, organized drawers and closets, cleaned house or did laundry today.

☐ I had 1-2-3 bowel movements today. I will drink a cup of warm lemon peel tea tonight before bed, if needed, to help with evacuation.

☐ Uplifting songs I played or sang today were:

_____

_____

Day 4

Today I may be almost free of craving carbohydrates. If cravings do come, I will eat a protein or fruit snack or drink some water until it passes because I may still have some deeper cleansing to do. I am remembering to be grateful. I continue to quickly forgive myself and others as impressions arise in my mind.

☐ I weighed _____ this morning.

☐ I got 6-7-8-9 hours of sleep last night.

☐ I ate breakfast.

☐ I took supplements: Vitamin/Mineral 1-2-3-4-5-6, Essential Fatty Acids (EFAs) 1-2-3-4, Digestive Enzymes 1-2-3-4-5-6, Ca/K/Mag 1-2-3-4, Extra B-Complex 1-2, Thermogenic Herbs 1-2-3-4-5-6, Probiotics 1-2-3, Cleansing Herbs 1-2-3-4, Other

_____

_____

_____

☐ Essential oils (EOs) I applied today were:

_____

_____

☐ I drank 1-2-3-4-5-6-7-8-9-10 glasses of pure water with *Lemon, Peppermint* or *Grapefruit* essential oils in several glasses.

☐ I ate 1-2-3 meal portions of lean protein today.

☐ I ate at least 1-2-3 portions of each vegetable category today; (green leafy), (green), (red, purple, & orange), (yellow & white) & (root veggies).

☐ I ate at the most 2 wholesome starches today, limiting brown rice, quinoa, oatmeal, winter squash, etc., to 1/4 cup and including whole grain bread and limiting all starches to about 100 calories.

☐ Today I measured out and used 1/4 to 1/2 teaspoon total of unrefined sea salt, for my day's ration of 1500 mg or less.

☐ I used fresh lemon juice and apple cider vinegar in salads or on food.

☐ I ate 1 or 2 apples or 1 or 2 small grapefruit today for snacks.

☐ I made 1-2 protein shake with water for snack today.

☐ I drank 1-2-3 cups of herb tea today: Green tea, Yerba Mate, Wu-Long Slimming Tea, Peppermint tea, and/or Chamomile tea.

☐ I did not eat any dairy products (cheese, cottage cheese) or deli meats, canned meats or pork products.

☐ I did not eat any condiments like mayonnaise, mustard, ketchup or any seasonings that contain salt or sugar.

☐ I did not drink any dairy products, fruit juices, sodas or sweet beverages, or more than 2 cups of coffee or regular black tea.

☐ I stretched, walked, did yoga, bounced on a mini-trampoline, or moved my lymph with a massage (w/out oil), or other form of exercise today

_____

_____

_____

☐ I took cleansing breath today and did some form of relaxation for stress relief: warm bath, dry skin brushing, meditation, laughed out loud, used essential oils.

☐ On a scale of 0 to 10 my energy was ____, my mood was ____, for sweet or salty foods, craving were ____, overall I felt ____.

☐ I reviewed or revised my food plans for the rest of the week to make sure I have everything I need of foods and spices.

☐ I had 1-2-3 bowel movements today. I drank a cup of warm lemon peel tea to help with cleansing.

☐ An inspiring thought I had today was:

_____

_____

_____

_____

Day 5

Today I am remembering that forgiveness is key to every aspect of my health.

☐ I weighed _____ this morning.

☐ I got 6-7-8-9 hours of sleep last night.

☐ I ate breakfast.

☐ I drank 1-2-3-4-5-6-7-8-9-10 glasses of pure water with *Lemon*, *Peppermint* or *Grapefruit* essential oils in some.

☐ I did not eat any dairy products (cheese, cottage cheese) or deli meats, canned meats or pork products.

☐ I took supplements: Vitamin/Mineral 1-2-3-4-5-6, Essential Fatty Acids (EFAs) 1-2-3-4, Digestive Enzymes 1-2-3-4-5-6, Ca/K/Mag 1-2-3-4, Extra B-Complex 1-2, Thermogenic Herbs 1-2-3-4-5-6, Probiotics 1-2-3, Cleansing Herbs 1-2-3-4,other

_____

_____

☐ EOs I applied today were:

_____

_____

☐ I ate 1-2-3 meal portions of lean protein today.

☐ I ate at least 1-2-3 portions of each vegetable category today; (green leafy), (green), (red, purple, & orange), (yellow & white) & (root veggies).

☐ I ate at the most 2 wholesome starches today, limiting brown rice, quinoa, oatmeal, winter squash, etc., to 1/4 cup and including whole grain bread and limiting all starches to 100 calories.

☐ Today I measured out and used 1/4 to 1/2 teaspoon total of unrefined sea salt for my day's ration of 1500 mg or less.

☐ I used fresh lemon juice and apple cider vinegar in salads or on food.

☐ I ate 1 or 2 apples or 1 or 2 small grapefruit today as snacks.

☐ I made 1-2 protein shake with water for snack today.

☐ I drank 1-2-3 cups of herb tea today: Green tea, Yerba Mate, Wu-Long Slimming Tea, Peppermint tea, and/or Chamomile tea.

☐ I did not eat any condiments like mayonnaise, mustard, ketchup or any seasonings that contain salt or sugar.

☐ I did not drink any dairy products, fruit juices, sodas or sweet beverages, or more than 2 cups of coffee or regular black tea.

☐ I stretched, walked, did yoga, mini-trampoline, or moved my lymph with a massage (w/out oil), or other form of exercise today

_____

_____

☐ I took cleansing breath today and did some form of relaxation for stress relief: warm bath, dry skin brushing, meditation, laughed out loud, used essential oils.

☐ On a scale of 0 to 10 my energy was ____, my mood was ____, for sweet or salty food cravings were ____, overall I felt ____.

☐ I reviewed or revised my food plans for the rest of the week to make sure I have everything I need.

☐ I had 1-2-3 bowel movements today. I drank a cup of lemon peel tea to help keep things moving along.

☐ I wrote a note or called a friend today to make plans to get-together.

Day 6

Today I will reflect on what I have learned about my reactions to food, and remember to apply this knowledge when I choose my meals.

☐ I weighed _____ this morning.

☐ I got 6-7-8-9 hours of sleep last night.

☐ I ate breakfast.

☐ I did not drink any dairy products, fruit juices, sodas or sweet beverages, or more than 2 cups of coffee or regular black tea.

☐ I ate at the most 2 wholesome starches today, limiting brown rice, quinoa, oatmeal, winter squash, etc., to 1/4 cup and including whole grain bread and limiting all starches to 100 calories.

☐ I did not eat any dairy products (cheese, cottage cheese) or deli meats, canned meats or pork products.

☐ I did not eat any condiments like mayonnaise, mustard, ketchup or any seasonings that contain salt or sugar.

☐ I ate at least 1-2-3 portions of each vegetable category today; (green leafy), (green), (red, purple, & orange), (yellow & white) & (root veggies).

☐ I took supplements: Vitamin/Mineral 1-2-3-4-5-6, Essential Fatty Acids (EFAs) 1-2-3-4, Digestive Enzymes 1-2-3-4-5-6, Ca/K/Mag 1-2-3-4, Extra B-Complex 1-2, Thermogenic Herbs 1-2-3-4-5-6, Probiotics 1-2-3, Cleansing Herbs 1-2-3-4, Other

_____

_____

☐ EOs I applied today were:

_____

_____

☐ I drank 1-2-3-4-5-6-7-8-9-10 glasses of pure water with *Lemon, Peppermint* or *Grapefruit* essential oils in some.

☐ I ate 1-2-3 meal portions of lean protein today.

☐ Today I measured out and used 1/4 to 1/2 teaspoon total of unrefined sea salt for my day's ration of 1500 mg or less.

☐ I used fresh lemon juice and apple cider vinegar in salads or on food.

☐ I ate 1 or 2 apples or 1 or 2 small grapefruit, or 1/2 an orange and/or 6 strawberries for a total of 2 fruit snacks today.

☐ I made 1-2 protein shake with water for snack today.

☐ I drank 1-2-3 cups of herb tea today: Green tea, Yerba Mate, Wu-Long Slimming Tea, Peppermint tea, and/or Chamomile tea.

☐ I stretched, walked, did yoga, mini-trampoline, or moved my lymph with a massage (w/out oil), or other form of exercise today

_____

_____

☐ I took cleansing breath today, and did some form of relaxation for stress relief: warm bath, dry skin brushing, meditation, laughed out loud, used essential oils.

☐ On a scale of 0 to 10 my energy was ____, my mood was ____, for sweet or salty, cravings were ____, overall I felt ____.

☐ I reviewed or revised my food plans for the rest of the week to make sure I have everything I need.

☐ I had 1-2-3 bowel movements today. I drank a cup of warm lemon peel tea to help with cleansing.

☐ I meditated, read, got fresh-air and sunshine, hugged someone, played a game, organized cabinets or desk, or did laundry today.

☐ I pray and meditate and count my blessings. Today I blessed others by:

_____

_____

_____

_____

_____

Day 7

Today I complete my first week eating a variety of colorful foods, lean protein and limited starches. I can choose to continue eating this way for the rest of my life, or when I feel ready I can commit to 3 weeks of the Rapid Weight Reduction plan.

☐ I weighed _____ this morning.

☐ I got 6-7-8-9 hours of sleep last night.

☐ I ate protein at breakfast.

☐ I took supplements: Vitamin/Mineral 1-2-3-4-5-6, Essential Fatty Acids (EFAs) 1-2-3-4, Digestive Enzymes 1-2-3-4-5-6, Ca/K/Mag 1-2-3-4, Extra B-Complex 1-2, Thermogenic Herbs 1-2-3-4-5-6, Probiotics 1-2-3, Cleansing Herbs 1-2-3-4, Other:

_____

☐ EOs I applied today were:

_____

☐ I drank 1-2-3-4-5-6-7-8-9-10 glasses of pure water with *Lemon, Peppermint* or *Grapefruit* essential oils in some.

☐ I ate 1-2-3 meal portions of lean protein today.

☐ I ate at least 1-2-3 portions of each vegetable category today; (green leafy), (green), (red, purple, & orange), (yellow & white) & (root veggies).

☐ I made 1-2 protein shake with water for snack today.

☐ I ate at most 2 wholesome starches today. 1 slice of bread was 50 calories or less.

☐ Today I measured out and used 1/4 to 1/2 teaspoon total of unrefined sea salt for my day's ration of 1500 mg or less.

☐ I used fresh lemon juice and apple cider vinegar in salads or on food.

☐ I ate 1 or 2 apples or 1 or 2 small grapefruit or 1/2 orange and/ or 6 strawberries for a total of two fruit snacks today.

☐ I drank 1-2-3 cups of herb tea today: Green tea, Yerba Mate, Wu-Long Slimming Tea, Peppermint tea, or Chamomile tea.

☐ I drink Yerba Mate or Green tea instead of coffee.

☐ I did not eat any dairy products (cheese, cottage cheese) or deli meats, canned meats or pork products.

☐ I did not eat any starchy carbs like rice, potatoes or pasta.

☐ I did not eat any condiments like mayonnaise, mustard, ketchup or any seasonings that contain salt or sugar.

☐ I did not drink any dairy products, fruit juices, sodas or sweet beverages, or more than 2 cups of coffee or regular black tea.

☐ I stretched, walked, did yoga, mini-trampoline, or moved my lymph with a massage (no oil), or other form of exercise today:

_____

_____

☐ I took cleansing breath today, and did some form of relaxation for stress relief: warm bath, dry skin brushing, meditation, laughed out loud, used essential oils.

☐ On a scale of 0 to 10 my energy was ____, my mood was ____, sweet or salty food cravings were ____, overall I felt ____.

☐ I reviewed or revised my food plans for the coming week.

☐ I had 1-2-3 bowel movements today. I drank a cup of warm lemon peel tea.

☐ My positive affirmation is:

_____

_____

☐ End of first week observations, and I am grateful for:

_____

_____

☐ Foods I noticed I feel good when I eat are:

_____

_____

☐ Foods I noticed I don't feel as well when I eat are:

_____

_____

_____

BODY AWARENESS

To enjoy lasting success with a lifestyle that depends on the vibrancy of nature's whole foods, we must also have conscious knowledge of the messages our bodies send to us, and be able to respond accordingly. One benefit of eating by the CMS plan is how sensitive you will become to the cues your body is giving you. You are not just retraining your palate to enjoy better dietary choices. You are learning which foods are best for your physiology by the way you feel after you've eaten them. This is especially so if you suspect you have certain food intolerances. You are learning to obey the hormone signals your body sends, such as when you are full and feeling nourished and satisfied so you stop eating or to recognize thirst signals when you are dehydrated and need to drink water instead of responding as if you were hungry instead of thirsty.

There is a good chance that these signals have become confused or you have ignored them for some time. Eating according to the CMS plan and using therapeutic-grade essential oils will help to re-establish order by clearing the receptor sites throughout the body systems. The innate wisdom of the body knows when it is being nourished and will repair imbalances and rebuild where necessary. If we expect to be well, we must consistently support our body's efforts.

There are all sorts of cues our bodies give us to bring our attention to imbalances. Pain is one you will recognize. That cue usually has a fairly loud volume, and it can be very insistent - with alarm bells - to get us to take notice. If ignored, the body still does the best it can for as long as it can by making adjustments here and there to cope with the inflamatory imbalance. The body always uses what it has available to do its best for us. It is far better when we are aware of shifts and changes in body systems energy, and know how to respond to the messages before a greater issue demands our attention. This awareness is also a key to becoming slimmer.

To this end, I have prepared some mini surveys as a way to help recognize any body systems that may be calling out to you. The more quickly you help relieve the stress of imbalance in your body systems, the more rapidly you will be able to reduce weight. This is a very simple place to start as an awareness exercise. Please consult with your health professionals if your body is sending you cues alerting you that medical attention may be needed.

In Section 8 you can review the many natural herbs, supplements and therapeutic-grade essential oils that have historically related to body systems' health. Your body just naturally knows how to use these gifts of nature.

COLOR ME SLIM & RAPID WEIGHT REDUCTION
Section 3: Table 1 - BASAL METABOLIC RATE

...Normal underarm morning temperature is 97.6 to 98.2.

...For every tenth of a point below 97.6 take 1 *Thyromin*.

...Example: 97.2 average temperature of 4 mornings = .4 below 97.6 = 4 capsules

...*Thyromin* may be taken in the morning for thyroid nutritional support.

... *Thyromin* may also be taken in the afternoon or at bedtime for adrenal and pituitary nutritional support and stress management.

BASAL METABOLIC RATE - A main function of our thyroid glands is to regulate metabolism. I did a little test to check my Basal Metabolic Rate (BMR). According to my average underarm temperature, my basal temperature was consistently low so I took the specific glandular nutrition of the Young Living formulation, *Thyromin*. I take it at bedtime or, if stressed, I take *Thyromin* in the morning for extra pituitary and adrenal support. Another nutritional formulation specific to the endocrine system I take especially when reducing weight is *EndoGize*. To be fair, I haven't done the BMR test again, but I'm more in tune to my body now.

You may wish to test yourself to learn if you have a low temperature first thing in the morning. Just know that this test is sensitive to certain conditions. If you sleep under an electric blanket or in an exceptionally warm room then your temperature would be influenced by this. You must be willing to lie still for at least ten minutes, and an old-fashioned glass thermometer works best. Take your body temperature four mornings in a row before getting up. The nights before testing shake down a glass thermometer to below 95 degrees and place it by the bed. Upon waking, carefully position the thermometer in your armpit. After ten minutes, record the temperature. Average four consecutive mornings. Basal body temperatures (BMR) below the range of 97.6 to 98.2 may reflect a lower rate of metabolism.

The essential oil blend I used to help create endocrine system balance, is *EndoFlex*. I place two drops over my throat or rubbed it into reflex points around the neck of my big toes. I now apply *Progessence Plus Serum* every day to help balance several symptoms related to low progesterone production - of which weight gain is one symptom.

WHEEL OF LIFE BALANCE

Section 3: Table 2 -

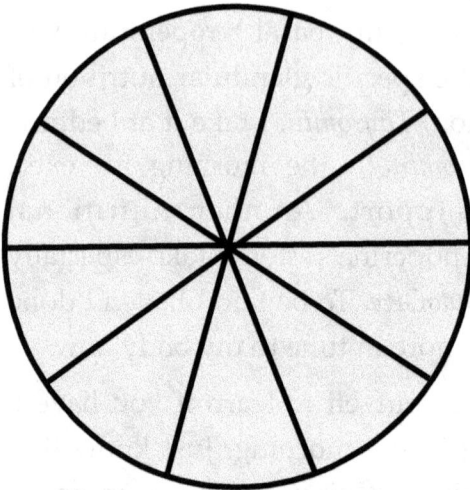

Label each of
the 10 sections
as follows:

1) SOCIAL LIFE   2) RELATIONSHIPS

3) HOME ENVIRONMENT   4) SPIRITUALITY

5) EDUCATION   6) FINANCES   7) CREATIVITY

8) CAREER   9) HEALTH   10) JOY & HUMOR

Mark each spoke with numerical values of 0 at the hub for the least satisfaction presently to 10 at the rim for greatest satisfaction at this time. Date your marks.

Connect the marks to reveal where greater balance may create a more rounded life.

Mark a new value on any spoke to indicate your goal to improve that area of your life.

Review monthly or quarterly, assess and date as your values and goals shift.

WHEEL OF FOOD BALANCE

Section 3: Table 3 -

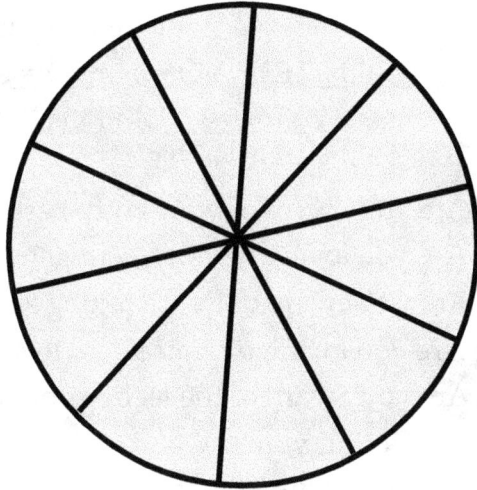

Label each of
the 10 sections
as follows:

1) COMPLETE PROTEIN   2) GREEN LEAFY VEGGIES

3) YELLOW, PALE GREEN, & WHITE VEGGIES

4) ROOT VEGGIES   5) GREEN VEGGIES   6) SEEDS & NUTS

7) RED, PURPLE, ORANGE VEGGIES   8) BEANS, PEAS & GRAINS

9) FRUITS & MELONS   10) QUALITY FATS & OILS

Place a mark to denote frequency of item eaten
as if 0 = not eaten at all, and 10 = eaten frequently.

0 is the value at the hub of the circle, and 10 is the
value at the rim of the circle.

Connect the marks to reveal present state of
dietary balance.

Improve consumption of less eaten categories to
provide yourself a well rounded variety of phytonutrients;
vitamins, minerals, enzymes & fiber.

SELF-AWARENESS SURVEY

Score each statement with the number that applies the most in the present.

<u>DEFINITELY NO = **1**   NO = **2**   NOT SURE = **3**</u>
<u>YES = **4**   DEFINITELY YES = **5**</u>

a.) Are you aware of your body parts?   _____

b.) Are you aware of your feelings?   _____

c.) Are you aware of the changing seasons?   _____

d.) Are you aware of your stress level?   _____

e.) Are you aware of the feelings of people
    around you?   _____

f.) Are you aware of tension in your muscles and back? _____

g.) Are you under too much stress?   _____

h.) Do you work with toxins?   _____

i.) Do you have trauma to your body often?   _____

j.) Do fungus, bacteria, or viruses cause you trouble?   _____

k.) Have sudden movements caused pain or
    discomfort?   _____

l.) Is your diet 40% or more fresh (not processed)
    food?   _____

m.) Do you eat a varied diet including all food
    groups?   _____

n.) Do you overeat or take megadoses of vitamins?   _____

o.) Do you eat processed foods or take
    synthetic vitamins?   _____

p.) Do you feel you digest, assimilate &
    eliminate your foods properly?   _____

If you have answered any question with a 3, indicating you are Not Sure, you may want to investigate that question to learn if you wish to become more fully aware in that area of your life.

Section 4

"I am the master of my fate;
I am captain of my soul."

~ Nelson Mandela

RAPID WEIGHT REDUCTION (RWR)

The subject of weight gain is a complex, many-sided issue that is presently a major discussion in the American culture. You know why this topic is so popular, and so very pressing. As mentioned before, research concludes that there is definitely a hypothalamus/weight gain connection, and growing evidence that points to digestive intolerance for gluten, many carbohydrate foods, and dairy sugars or protein.

The Color Me Slim Plan for Rapid Weight Reduction (RWR) is the plan I developed and implemented for myself. For years I thought of myself as one who ate a fairly healthy diet, but you would not know it by the weight I had gained during those years. I believe now that the culprit has a name: Carbohydrate Intolerance (CI).

When I realized that most people would not be able to jump feet-first into the RWR plan without some preparation, I adapted the basic Color Me Slim plan as a place to start and a place to "rest" between the more rigorous three weeks of RWR cycles. Even though these plans are presented here, drawing on my background and experience, know that they are still works in progress.

There are no special considerations of other valid approaches of dieting by blood type, body type or metabolic type. It is, however, what I did using the Young Living products for cleansing, rebuilding, and supporting nutrition and stress-release. I am a living testimony to the quality and effectiveness of the Young Living products as they helped to give me the strength and courage to believe I could accomplish this personal paradigm shift after so many years of "dabbling" with the intention to change my attitude and diet.

Perhaps you have also been looking for an all-natural plan of eating fresh, easy-to-fix whole foods without having to depend on prepackaged, expensive meals. It is true that I promote eating high-quality, organically farmed foods. It is also true that these foods can cost more than commercially raised versions, but I think you will find that organically grown foods not only taste better, but are free of herbicide and pesticide toxins that you do not want burdening your glands among other tissues. Also, by not buying the items on the restricted list, you will be redirecting those grocery dollars for greater health by eating organic, free-range and grass-fed more often. May I suggest that you seriously consider the real cost of fast-foods, chips, sugary snacks and drinks and "empty calorie" foods you may be presently buying? Repurposing those dollars to natural, whole foods, essential oils and supplements will definitely offset some of the expense of your new program. (I also like to think that we are not paying doctor bills we probably would otherwise have experienced.)

If you choose two, three or four things to eliminate (hopefully sugar will be first to go) or add healthier foods by slowly adapting some of the CMS ideas to create new habits, implementing the Rapid Weight Reduction (RWR) plan will not be a shock, but it will require concentrated effort of all aspects of the plan. You will not, and must not, go hungry.

On RWR you will very carefully choose totally healthy foods while eliminating the restricted items. This should not cause illness or undue distress. However, it is always wise to consult with your doctor to be well informed of any reason you should adjust your diet and/or exercise according to your personal circumstances. Additionally, if at any time you feel RWR is too much for you, just discontinue it and return to the gentle ease of CMS until you feel ready again. Remember, you are the one in control of your health.

RAPID WEIGHT REDUCTION

Section 4: Table 1 - RWR BASICS

• Eat 3 colorful, balanced meals daily.

• Eat certain allowable fruits & protein snacks daily.

• No missed meals.

• Eliminate sugar, most grains & starch foods for 3 weeks.

• Limit good fats to 2 tablespoons per day.

• Identify and avoid toxic foods & chemicals.

• Get quality rest & reduce stress.

• Promote endocrine system functional nutrition.

• Promote thyroid health. Use natural oral care such as Young Living's *Thieves* products.

• Use natural skin & hair care. Limit creams & vegetable oil based lotions & cosmetics. Do not use products containing mineral oil on your skin.

FOOD INTOLERANCE

You may adjust the RWR plan to spend the first two weeks of Rapid Weight Reduction as a time to test yourself to learn if you may have some intolerance to digesting the starches and sugars of carbohydrates (Carbohydrate Intolerance or CI), gluten intolerance or perhaps some dairy lactose or casein intolerance. To do this, it would be wise to work with a qualified health care practitioner.

You will be totally avoiding all forms of sugars, grains or dairy. An internet search will reveal some ideas of what is involved to be sure to have valid, reliable results.

YOUNG LIVING ESSENTIAL OILS
Section 4: Table 2 - ESSENTIAL OILS & RWR

Frankincense, Gathering, Grounding, Harmony, Inspiration, Sacred Mountain, Sandalwood
for Centering, Grounding, Meditation & Prayer

Di-Gize & Peppermint for Digestive System Support

Stress Away Roll-On & RutaVaLa for Stress Release

Grapefruit to Help Dissolve Fat & Cellulite

Lemon for Lymph System Support

Thieves for Immune System Support

Valor for Energy Balancing

FOUR WEEKS FOR RAPID WEIGHT REDUCTION

This Rapid Weight Reduction (RWR) plan is taken one week at a time for four consecutive weeks:

Week 1 - On CMS, Preparing for RWR

Week 2 - Begin RWR

Week 3 - On RWR, making adjustments

Week 4 - End RWR, measure and assess

You will notice that RWR allows a generous amount of food that must be eaten in Week 1. That's right! You will not be deprived, and while you are filling yourself with volumes of allowable foods, you will be busy with the logistics of preparing for the next 3 weeks of strict adherence to RWR.

On RWR you will be very mindful of when, how and what you eat. I emphasize the "rules" as strict and must be faithfully followed for the next three weeks because it is the way you will learn which foods from the RWR lists work the best for you by encouraging your body to use stored fat for energy. If you are not precisely following the plan, you may miss the subtle signs and messages telling you to notice how you feel from that meal. When a meal is very satisfying, and you've digested it well and feel nourished, then you have created good chemistry in your body's laboratory that you will want to repeat time-and-again for weight reduction and to help with maintenance later. So to begin, stay with the plan by holding the attitude that you are making the efforts to listen to your body while it is restoring balance, especially to hypothalamus and digestive functions. May this month be a happy start toward that end.

Week 1 - PREPARATION FOR RWR

- Continue to follow the basic CMS plan as long as it takes to regulate your bowels to prepare your body for rapid fat removal.

- Focus on kidney and liver cleansing to ready these organs for increased activity. (I used one bottle of Young Living's *K&B Tincture* during this prep time.)

- If you have not already tracked your Metabolic Basal Temperature or have this knowledge from tests your doctor has ordered of a thyroid assessment, do it this week. (See instructions in Section 3.)

- When your bowels are moving well every day, it is a good indication you should be able to move into RWR. If you did not use Young Living's *Rhemogen Tincture* on CMS, I would do it now and continue throughout the 3 weeks or until the bottle is empty.

- After your prep stage of 3 days (up to a week or more if necessary), when you are no longer eating any foods from the restricted list, move into RWR to train your body to use stored fat to fuel your energy.

- Drink the required amount of pure water, which is 1/2 your weight in ounces. (See important water information in Section 7.)

- Eating out should be held to a minimum for these 3 weeks. It can be done, but take care and don't make it a habit. Take a pass on all buffet type establishments.

- Getting plenty of rest, some sunshine, and fresh air and light exercise is recommended. Use Young Living's *Progesessence Plus Serum* (women only),

RutaVaLa Roll-On, Peace & Calming and/or *Lavender* essential oil before bed.

- De-stress, laugh, sing, dance, watch funny movies, visit a comedy club, soak in the tub with *Lavender* essential oils, meditate. Use Young Living's *Valor, Stress Away,* and *Relaxation Roll-On* essential oils as a convenient way to consistently send calming energy to the hypothalamus for better appetite control, reset satiety messages and re-establish a higher metabolism set-point.

Week 1 is a busy week. Arrange your schedule to accomplish the following:

1. Prepare the Daily Journal worksheets again by taking your "before" pictures and measurements. Now that you are familiar with the Daily Journal worksheets, you can make copies, add to my list or make up your own. It is VERY important that you keep the Journal current.

2. Complete the surveys to have a baseline of tracking.

3. Assess yourself and write down all your body cues, signs and symptoms.

4. Get clarity about cleansing to prepare for RWR, and what must be done for the first few days to achieve regular bowel movements.

5. Start drinking herb teas and/or warm lemon juice tea the very first day for cleansing. (Squeeze the juice of 1/2 organic lemon into 1 cup of warm water.)

6. Begin to measure water to be sure you are drinking at least 1/2 of your weight in ounces.

7. Consult the checklist of foods, and make a shopping list to be able to prepare several meals. For the first three days you should eat unlimited amounts of lean meats, 2 eggs every morning and plenty of uncooked salads and vegetables. Eat raw fruits, vegetables, nuts and seeds for the first 3 days. Cook meats and eggs.

8. Begin eating unlimited amounts of food from the RWR food lists to stimulate a thermogenic response and help cleansing.

9. Do not eat starchy carbs, sugars, sodium, or caffeine.

10. Decide teas, supplements, and essential oil products you will order. Place orders to have products delivered by the start of week 2. (See Sections 8 & 9 for Young Living.)

11. Clear and clean your refrigerator and pantry. Now is a good time to use only "green" products if you are not yet doing so.

12. Take inventory again for your shopping list.

13. Pitch or pack away any food items that are sure to tempt.

14. Prepare a big sign with a question mark on it to put on your refrigerator to help remind you of your *why* and to ask yourself, "What is my best choice?"

15. Ask for family support and tell at least two close friends or family members your plans and your goals for the next month.

16. Visit your doctor to request to be monitored, and to have records of blood work, etc. (It is part of the adventure to see how your numbers improve.)

17. Arrange your schedule to have the time needed to learn and practice this eating plan.

18. Decide the form(s) of exercise you want to do, and get any clothing or equipment that will help ensure you exercise.

19. Decide on recipes for meals and snacks for several days to have the fresh ingredients ready when needed.

20. Review the lists of foods and chemicals to avoid at www.ewg.com, Environmental Working Group's website.

21. Seriously curtail *or eliminate* the use of vegetable oils, creams and lotions on your skin since they must be handled by your body like other fats. Instead you want your body to learn to draw on the stored fat as energy fuel - not oil-based chemical concoctions.

22. Start spending some stress-release time and learn how therapeutic-grade essential oils help relieve stress.

23. Start soaking in Epsom Salts and baking soda baths (equal portions, 1:1) with *Lavender* essential oils to help release toxins and for deep relaxation. I like to add about 5-8 drops of *Geranium* essential oil too.

24. Schedule dry massage (without oils) to help move lymph fluids, release muscle tension, etc.

25. Be prayerful and grateful.

26. Take this first week to figure out how to do RWR and decide some of the better ways things will work going forward.

27. Don't forget to weigh yourself every morning and faithfully mark your Daily Journal for tracking. Don't obsess, weighing only once a day around the same time each day is enough.

The first week of CMS is the prep portion of RWR, and it is very important to use this week to focus on establishing regular elimination habits. Since you decided to start eating this way, are you beginning to feel any differently? Cravings should get easier now that you are drinking plenty of water and flushing out sugar residue.

YOUNG LIVING ESSENTIAL OILS
Section 4: Table 3 - RWR NUTRITIONAL PRODUCTS

CHOOSE FROM AMONG THESE 8 PRODUCTS FOR WEEK ONE*

ComforTone	Peace & Calming Essential Oil
K&B Tincture	Rehemogen Tincture
Lavender Essential Oil	RutaVaLa Roll-On
Omega Blue EFAs	Super B

OTHER SUPPORTIVE PRODUCTS TO CONSIDER

Balance Complete	
Dentarome Toothpaste	Progessence Plus Serum
Di-Gize Essential Oil Blend	Pure Protein Complete
Endogize	Stress Away Roll-On
Essentialzyme	SuperCal
Life 5 Probiotic	ThermaBurn
MultiGreens	Thyromin
NingXia Red	True Source

*Note that the lists throughout this book reflect the names of products I have used over the course of many years to gain and maintain balance. The lists reveal the variety of Young Living products avilable as support for healthy body systems.

Once you decide that your body is cleansing well enough, you should be ready to move into the rapid reduction, RWR, three-week plan. Do the starchy foods and fruit snacks agree with you, or do you suspect you do not tolerate them well because of bloating, sleepiness after eating, etcetera? If so, you may wish to test yourself by making a few adjustments to the RWR plan for at least two weeks so you can find the diet most appropriate for you.

YOUNG LIVING ESSENTIAL OILS
Section 4: Table 4 - RWR NUTRITIONAL PRODUCTS

YOU MAY CHOOSE FROM AMONG THESE PRODUCTS
FOR
WEEK TWO & BEYOND

Cleansing & Building: *ComforTone, Digest+Cleanse, InnerDefense, K&B Tincture, ICP Fiber, Life 5 Probiotics, Rehemogen Tincture*

Digestion: *Detoxzyme, Di-Gize EO, Essentialzyme, GLF EO, JuvaCleanse, JuvaPower, JuvaSpice, JuvaTone, Life 5 Probiotics, Peppermint EO*

Essential Oils: *Di-Gize, EndoFlex, Grapefruit, Lavender, Lemon, Peppermint, Purification, Stress Away or Tranquil or RutaVaLa Roll-On, Thieves, Valor*

Glandular Support: *Cortistop, Endogize, PD 80/20, ProGen, Progessence Plus Serum, Stevia Extract, Thyromin, Women's Cortistop*

Nutritional: *Balance Complete, Master Formula Hers/His, Mega Cal, Mineral Essence, MultiGreens, NingXia Red, Omega Blue EFAs, Power Meal, Pure Protein Complete, SuperB, Super C, Super Cal, True Source*

Personal Care: *ART Skin Care, Hair Care, Lotions & Skin Creams, Thieves Oral Care*

Thermogenics: *ThermaBurn, Ultra Young Plus Oral Spray*

Week 2 - ON THE PLAN

Ready to move into RWR? Remember the rules must be followed for best results. If you happen to stray at any time just get back on the plan soon, but know that these rules are not to be thought of as punitive. They're designed to build momentum. You will lose momentum each time you stray for the next three weeks - especially with fructose and sugar. It takes about two weeks for the liver to begin to regenerate.[17] If you begin to eliminate excitotoxins then go back to eating fake, sugar-laden or high fructose corn syrup foods, you take the chance of a set back.

To give you more insight that might be useful to you, I especially took note of my weight the morning of the start of my second week. I had already dropped some weight, but this would now be my new baseline number. I had learned that weighing myself at about the same time every morning just after I emptied my bladder would be my guide to help me gauge how I was doing. I could immediately see the next day if my body started retaining fluid or was reacting adversely to what I'd eaten or to activities from the day before, so I could make immediate adjustments.

Try tracking your weight by weighing yourself each morning. Use your scales as a tool to help recognize if certain foods or environmental factors cause fluid retention, and use the scales to cheer yourself on too. Don't get upset any morning it appears you have gained. THIS IS GOING TO HAPPEN! It is normal for your weight to fluctuate a pound or more, but if it should happen that your weight goes up by as much as 2 pounds, you'll know to turn the trend around by being very careful about your plan. It is this one little trick of weight awareness that can help you maintain a healthy weight for the rest of your life, but you definitely don't want it to become obsessive. Only weigh once each day. The goal isn't to lose weight to no end, but to reach a healthy, stable weight, and to see that reflected in the scale.

Another key trick that has helped me maintain my weight I learned from Dr. Batmanghelidj's book, Your Body's Many Cries for Water - You Are Not Sick, You Are Thirsty!, is to faithfully measure out my drinking water at 1/2 my weight in ounces each day. I avoid iced drinks since they slow digestion and increase hunger, and I often put a drop or two of *Lemon, Grapefruit* or *Peppermint* essential oil in my water. To avoid the possibility that taking in this much water could flush valuable nutrients, I take Young Living's *SuperCal* to supply calcium, magnesium and potassium throughout the day. I used to have leg cramps and restless leg at night which are body signals for poor hydration and possibly the need for more potassium. These symptoms no longer arise since I stay hydrated with plenty of water and take a *SuperCal* at each meal about six days a week. A tip for office workers is to keep a bottle of drinking water near the restroom and make it a habit to drink a big glass after each rest break.

This new diet is destined to become new blood, bone and flesh. With my plan I was able to both cleanse and build at the same time. Which, by the way, is what nature intends for our diets to do.

Remember, the underlying goal is to return glandular function from the chaos that old patterns have created. Learn the rules of new habits that support your glands and weight management and the old habits soon diminish. Thermogenic foods and herbs such as Young Living's *ThermaBurn* will help with this. *ThermaBurn* is a weight control herbal complex with thermogenic essential oils that help curb appetite, raise metabolism, boost energy, and combat fatigue for enhanced weight management. It contains liver cleansers and de-fattening factors to increase metabolism. This supplement helped me to clear cravings in the first week, and I consumed one bottle of *ThermaBurn* while concentrating on the three weeks of rapid weight reduction.

Beginning with the basic color categories of vegetables, and comparing the Glycemic Index of foods and other values listed about each of the foods, I chose the foundational nutrition necessary to maintain my health during rapid weight reduction. I include fruits for snacks (those lower on the Glycemic Index), and nuts and sprouted seeds in limited quantities for healthy fats.

Prepare each day's meals from this RWR Food List. Do not skip meals. Carry snacks and water with you.

Choose items from each vegetable category as follows:

- Green Leafy - turnip greens, spinach, beet greens, collard greens, Romaine lettuce, cilantro, kale, parsley, cabbage, Swiss chard, watercress. Eat cabbage and mustard greens sparingly until off of RWR since they are thought to interfere somewhat with the uptake of iodine.

- Red, Orange & Purple - red bell pepper, pimento peppers, egg plant (limit), purple cabbage, pumpkin (limit), acorn squash, tomatoes, yams (limit).

- Pale Yellow & Green, Yellow or White - yellow summer squash, green onions, bean sprouts, cauliflower, celery, cucumbers, endive, garlic, leeks, mushrooms, water chestnuts, zucchini.

- Green - artichoke (limit), asparagus, broccoli, Brussels sprouts, okra, green bell peppers, snow or snap peas, string beans - no English peas.

- Root - carrots (limit), radishes, turnips, potatoes (limit), onions, garlic, kohlrabi, sweet potatoes (limit) or yams (limit).

Choose eggs, lean meats or fish for 3 meals each day as follows:

- eggs - 1 egg (or 2 if 1 becomes a protein snack) per day fixed any style except fried. True free-range/cage-free, fresh eggs are greatly preferred.

- beef & bison - 4 ounces raw weight, choose lean cuts, trim the fat, drain fat as you cook, don't fry, eat only 2 X per week, never on the same day, and skip at least one day between beef meals. Organic, grass-fed preferred.

- chicken & turkey - 6 ounces raw weight, skinless, white meat, baked, broiled, grilled, stewed, no frying, no gravy. True free-range, organic preferred.

- lamb & mutton - 4-5 ounces raw weight, lean chops, baked, grilled.

- fish - 5-6 ounces raw weight of any sea food of choice except salmon, 4 ounces, baked, broiled, grilled and canned tuna 4 ounces. (Limit shell fish.)

Choose from only these fruits as follows:

- apples - 1 medium or 2 small apples AND...

- grapefruit -1 medium grapefruit or 1/2 large OR...

- orange - 1 orange split 1/2 for 2 different snacks OR...
- strawberries - 6 strawberries medium size (only if needed for variety).
- lemon - 1 lemon per day if you tolerate lemon.

LIMIT OR AVOID GRAINS WHILE ON RWR as follows:

- barley - bread or cereal (limit).
- buckwheat - 1/4 C hot cereal, thermogenic for winter months, (limit).
- corn - no corn, corn products, corn meal or corn starch.
- millet - limit as it is thought to hinder iodine uptake by the thyroid.
- oats - organic rolled oats 1/4 C (limit gluten, eat only if you desire starch variety).
- rye - bread or crackers 50 calorie or less, crackers - calculate calories to adjust amount.
- rice - organic long grain brown rice, 1/4 cup as starch serving, (limit).
- spelt - bread 50 calorie or less, may need to divide a slice that is higher in calories.
- quinoa - 1/4 C cooked as starch serving (limit).
- whole wheat - eat only in sprouted grain bread, avoid when testing for CI and gluten intolerance.

Choose fats & oils as follows:

- Good fats are needed for successful weight reduction. Choose Better Butter (See recipe Section 6), Organic Virgin Olive Oil or Organic Coconut Oil.

- Limit all fats to minimal amount each day - 2 TBS total, at the most, on RWR.

- Do not eat cheese for the 3 weeks of RWR, and no nut butters on RWR.

- Supplement with Essential Fatty Acids (EFAs) such as Young Living's *Omega Blue*.

Choose condiments as follows:

- Use fresh or dried herbs for seasoning, apple cider vinegar, red wine vinegar, unrefined sea salt, (limit to 1/4 to 1/2 tsp per day), liquid aminos (limit), supplement with herbal stevia, garlic and onion powders, lemon juice.

- No catsup, mayonnaise, or pickles.

Drink pure water or filtered at home (preferably in non-plastic bottles).

- Seek and use the cleanest source of non-chlorinated water to drink and bathe. Drink 1/2 your body weight in ounces daily.

- Flavor water with a drop of *Grapefruit, Lemon,* or *Peppermint* essential oils.

Drink herb teas as follows:

- Drink at least 1 cup herb tea (Green, Yerba Mate, or Wu Long Chinese Slimming Tea every day), Peppermint tea as digestive aid, Chamomile to relax and rest.

- Drink Green tea if hungry.

- Drink Parsley Tea for potassium balance when sodium causes fluid retention or if legs cramp.

> ▸ Drink Lemon Peel Tea to help elimination.

You may supplement with products you already have for body systems support. The point is to give your body the nutritional elements it needs to accomplish your wellness and weight reduction goals.

Week 3 - MAKING ADJUSTMENTS

Now that you've had a full week of living with a totally whole food plan, and all prepackaged convenience foods are no longer part of your menu planning, it really isn't so bad, is it? Is there any part of the plan that is particularly difficult for you to follow? Is RWR too aggressive and too ambitious for you right now? If so, perhaps you would like to drop back to the CMS plan until you feel ready to fully commit to RWR at another time. That is just fine.

Please don't get so discouraged that you totally give up. Working with CMS, you can still gradually cleanse your body and environment by avoiding toxins and becoming more familiar with the benefits of the therapeutic-grade essential oils. However, one caution - it really is important to eliminate refined sugars because of the endocrine and immune system imbalances they cause.

Do you think you could muster the courage to try for just one more week? You'll be almost through the first month, and then the last week of RWR seems easier.

I found I was able to pick right up where I left off after just a brief rest from the strictness of RWR, and it was even easier the second time around because I truly did eliminate the sugars and ate only limited amounts of starchy foods.

Are you exercising? Exercise helps to move the toxins out more quickly. This brings our attention to the idea of having a colonic irrigation done by a professional therapist. Colonics are the best way I know of to quickly eliminate toxins, perhaps parasites, and old encrusted material that could be lining the colon wall and inhibiting absorption of nutrients. Believe it or not, I found this to be a very relaxing process, and psychologically I just knew that I was giving my body a better chance at getting rid of acids and poisons. Besides, when I think that 80% of my immune system is in the colon, I get real clear about my intention to cleanse and build.

Did you know that every cell of our bodies has four basic necessities, and we can influence the level or quality at which these four necessities take place by our diets and supplementation? They are:

1. HYDRATION - Living organisms can't live without water.

2. OXYGEN - Living organisms can't live without air.

3. NUTRITION - The body will do the best it can for as long as it can with what we give to it. It's far better if we provide quality nutrition.

4. ELIMINATION - Every cell needs to be able to expel and be rid of its metabolic waste products.

Do you see how CMS and RWR are designed to facilitate these four basic cellular needs? As you enter this third week of RWR, think about the preventive steps you are taking. Good for you! I'm sure you realize how important it is to follow on or you would not have come this far.

Use your essential oils, <u>don't skip meals</u>, <u>get plenty of restful sleep</u>, <u>and eat snacks</u> to keep your blood sugar and metabolism running smoothly. Drink water and herb teas.

Week 4 - MEASURE AND ASSESS

You've been eating only colorful, live foods, drinking plenty of purified water, listening to the messages your body sends about certain foods or combinations of foods and have been eliminating regularly. You've avoided the foods that are either high on the Glycemic Index or on the Foods to Avoid list compiled by the Environmental Working Group because of chemical toxins that interfere with your body systems' functions. (See Web Reference, Section 10.)

By now you should have measurable results to report. At the end of the fourth week or first month, perform all the measurements and assessments again, recording your results. No doubt congratulations are in order.

You've come a good way toward cleansing and providing the raw materials for your body to build new blood, nerves and tissues. Do you have a plan for moving forward? Is the reason you were inspired or determined to make these changes still motivating you? Take care for the following two weeks to gradually add back the starches, nuts and fruits you were not eating on RWR.

By consistently providing quality nutrients and cleansing, your blood cells can be transformed to greater health every 90 days. Make a personal commitment to cycle through RWR at least two more times after resting two weeks between cycles with CMS. Experience the difference new blood cells make in vigor and immunity.

Though the basic CMS plan is somewhat more lenient than RWR, it is still a healthy way to eat and live. After this first month on RWR, you should know which foods your body seems to prefer and those that are more difficult for you. You can return to the CMS plan for as long as you wish. If you were not able to completely avoid or eliminate everything suggested on the RWR list, perhaps you will choose to concentrate on one or two more of these now.

Complete the one month measurement record. Do the same for each month thereafter, and maintain your Daily Journal Worksheets.

We invite you to share your experiences with us. Visit our web site often (www.ColorMeSlim.com), and register for our CMS e-news to receive notice of upcoming web-based sessions. Please post your comments, support others, and look for help from the community of "sweet people" on our blog.

Our E-mail is info@ColorMeSlim.com.

COLOR ME SLIM/RWR
MEASUREMENTS - END OF 4 WEEKS

Name _____ Date_____

    Stand before a mirror. If you choose to wear clothes, wear the same clothing each time you measure. Compare values with beginning measurements.

    I weighed _____ this morning. Body fat was_____% Hydration was_____%.

❖ My chest measurement is _____.

Measure the chest at nipple level.

❖ My waist measurement is _____.

Bend to the side, measure waist at crease.

❖ My lower abs measurement is _____.

Measured at the widest spot or about 2" below the navel.

❖ My hips measure _____.

Hips are measured at the widest area around.

❖ My thighs measure _____ R _____ L

Mark thighs about 9" above each knee then measure around.

❖ My calves measure _____ R _____ L

Calves are measured at about mid-calf while standing.

❖ My upper arms measure _____ R _____ L

Upper arms are measured at about mid-arm.

❖ I now wear a size _____ shirt/blouse & size _____ pants.

❖ My blood pressure is _____/_____.

    Some grocery stores and drug stores have complimentary blood pressure stations or you can buy a small unit to use at home.

94

WEEK 5 & BEYOND

Here's a simple plan for the next 8 weeks to complete your 3 months or 90 days of healthy eating and stress reduction:

Weeks 5 and 6, Balancing and Maintaining - You are returning to CMS and resting from RWR for at least two weeks. You no longer need to observe the directions for the first 3 days of Week 1 on CMS. You've already done that, so just continue on CMS for weeks 5 and 6 as a rest period between the more aggressive weight reduction of RWR.

Weeks 7 through 9, RWR - Measure and assess at end of week 9 (2 months).

Weeks 10 through 12, (like week 5) Balancing and Maintaing - End of 12 weeks (3 months), measure and assess. Just think; stronger blood, bone and nerve tissue!

Did you make a 90-day personal commitment? Congratulations! Rest from the RWR plan for at least 2 weeks before you initiate it again, should you wish to do so.

CMS & RWR
Section 4: Table 5 - MAINTAINING BALANCE

- Continue eating protein & choosing veggies from each category every day.
- Remember to eat at least one item from each food category to receive the food values of all the colors every day.
- Introduce new foods into your diet to add variety.
- Avoid sugar & stimulants.
- Limit breads, bakery goods & starchy grains.
- Drink plenty of pure water flavored with therapeutic-grade essential oils.
- Be grateful, stretch & relax.
- Find humor in everyday life. Laugh out loud!

HELPING OTHERS - Are you considering sharing this program with someone? Would you like to know how you can help others with this great need facing our country today, and satisfy financial needs as well? Tell the person who shared this book with you about your growing interest in all that Young Living has to offer.

Each Young Living product not only delivers a bounty of nutritional factors, but they also carry a certain purchase value that creates income for Independent Distributors who refer others to the company. Therefore, another great need facing many in our world is addressed through Young Living's marketing plan too.

There are so many advantages to becoming involved with Young Living that reach beyond the benefits the supplements, skin care and essential oils offer. Such as:

- ❖ Social interaction, travel/trips, peer recognition.
- ❖ Business-building, entrepreneurship with pertinent helps and tools, educational opportunities.
- ❖ Fulfilling your purpose - personal growth.
- ❖ Be a leader and mentor - business and product training.
- ❖ Engage in "green" initiatives for personal reasons and the greater environment.
- ❖ Receive compensation for referrals in a global market, no matter where you choose to do business.
- ❖ Cover the cost of your family's product usage.
- ❖ Financial freedom - structure for long-term, residual income - free up discretionary time - more family time and carefree fun with friends and family.
- ❖ Enjoy business tax advantages.

Section 5

" Adopt the pace of nature:
her secret is patience."

~ Ralph Waldo Emerson

CLEANSING HABITS

As mentioned, an absolute MUST to release fat from the body is to make sure the bowels are evacuating every day - hopefully more than once a day. If this is not happening for you, the Young Living cleansing products can assist with this important priority. Each person starting RWR will do well to aid cleansing of the blood and colon. *Rhemogen Tincture* from Young Living is a gentle-acting liquid concentration of herbs and essential oils like Cascara sagrada bark, *Melaleuca, Thyme* and other natural ingredients that enhance elimination and have been historically known for their internal cleansing and building properties. As Dr. Bernard Jensen taught, "Life and death are in the colon... the blood is only as clean as the colon."[18]

Changing your diet can often cause constipation. If you are already constipated when you begin RWR, then it will be a high priority to address the proper functioning of this body system. The modern lifestyle is linked to bowel disorders like constipation as the accumulation of ingested "toxic substances like pesticides, additives, preservatives, sweeteners, food dyes, bleaches, synthetic flavor enhancers, drinking and bathing in chlorinated water, metals, drugs, and other chemicals"[19] are hanging out in our colons or fat cells. Even pharmaceuticals such as antibiotics create internal imbalance by destroying the "good" gut bacteria along with the "bad."

Adhering to RWR will ensure that you will be greatly limiting the addition of these toxins while releasing them from storage in your fat cells and other tissues. Fat cells are little sacs that become plump as they hold toxins away from vital organs until we have the energetic integrity to cleanse.

As we are able to safely release the toxins into our colon for elimination or through the skin with perspiration, our fat cells shrink (this is one way we become slimmer), but they are still there ready to plump up again if the fat is not used as fuel. Consequently, you can see how important it is to keep the colon open for the detoxification process to complete its cycles of elimination without having the unfortunate circumstance of redepositing the toxins again into the fat cells.

You can start gently with *Rehemogen Tincture* and *ComforTone* to help the evacuation of accumulated wastes, but also to keep the colon able to receive the toxins cleansed from the fat cells as a result of eating the RWR diet. One bottle of *Rehemogen Tincture* may be all you will need when you start RWR, but this is one product I like to have on the shelf all the time, as well as *ComforTone* capsules. These may be taken along with warm, cleansing Lemon Peel Tea (See instructions, Section 5: Table 1, page 105.) or special herb teas found at health food stores.

As much as 80% of your immune system is in the colon. "Friendly bacteria" colonies live here to do the work of detoxifying and purifying in this very hostile environment. This bowel flora must be encouraged to proliferate, implant and grow to help us maintain a healthy immune system. If there is an overgrowth of the unfriendly microorganisms such as yeasts (like candida albicans), the bowel wall can become weakened and these yeasts can escape the bowel through a leaky gut to become a systemic problem. Yeast and fungus problems such as candida and athletes foot indicate an overgrowth of these micro-organisms. Eating plain (no fruit or sugar) Greek Yogurt and drinking plain kefir will assist your body in restoring essential gut bacteria as well as taking Young Living's *Life 5*.

Weight reduction will be hampered and more difficult if there is an overgrowth of unfriendly bacteria in our bodies. Do you crave sugar, breads or alcoholic beverages? Do tobacco smoke or strong fragrances really bother you? If so, suspect yeast overgrowth. On the RWR plan, it is most important to ensure that your friendly bacteria is at peak performance to help combat any yeast overgrowth. Supplementation with a probiotic will not only assist in this way, but probiotics are also known to help with minor digestive discomforts and support immune function. Probiotic literally means "pro-life."

Taking Young Living's *Life 5* probiotic formulation is a first-line-of-defense product that will facilitate RWR. Also, to create an unfriendly environment for harmful yeast and fungus, Young Living's *Inner Defense* is a powerhouse of therapeutic-grade essential oils known for their purifying effects. Should my family need to addresses fungal and yeast overgrowth, we would support our immune systems with *Inner Defense* and apply *Thieves* blend essential oils to the bottoms of our feet morning and night and use *Oregano* essential oil on our feet and toes.

RWR is a pro-life plan that starts with gentle cleansing and gradually goes on to help the body be rid of toxins at deeper and deeper levels. All body systems will function better and the threat of serious organ dysfunction and health problems that could require medical attention may be averted. For best results, I suggest 3 cycles of RWR as major segments or at least a 90-day program completed each year.

It's possible to relieve stress and release toxins by soaking in a tub with essential oils (e.g., *Lavender* and *Geranium*, 5-8 drops each) in Epsom Salts (magnesium salts) and baking soda (1:1). Another help is to gently do Dry Skin Brushing all over the body to exfoliate and increase the skin's efficiency in releasing toxins - it is our "third kidney" after all. As your body is freed from harmful toxins, fungus, yeast, parasites and excess fecal matter, you will be reducing weight along with these toxic energetic drains, and that's when you will begin to experience the rewards of true health.

YOUNG LIVING ESSENTIAL OILS
Section 5: Table 1 -
CLEANSING HABITS

PRODUCTS THAT SUPPORT ELIMINATIVE SYSTEMS

5-Day Nutritive Cleanse

Cleansing Trio

ComforTone Capsules

Digest+Cleanse

Essentialzyme

I.C.P. Fiber Blend

Inner Defense

Di-Gize Essential Oil Blend

K & B Tincture

Life 5 Probiotic

Rhemogen Tincture

YOUNG LIVING ESSENTIAL OILS
Section 5: Table 2 -
LOVE YOUR LIVER

PRODUCTS THAT SUPPORT THE LIVER

GLF, & JuvaCleanse essential oil blends (powerful)

JuvaFlex & Release essential oil blends (alternate application sites over liver & foot reflex points)

JuvaPower & Juva Spice nutritionals (mix in smoothies & replace salt)

JuvaTone nutritional supplement (cleanse & build)

Lemon and *Grapefruit* essential oils (emulsify fats)

Omega Blue Essential Fatty Acids (with essential oils)

Rhemogen Tincture (blood cleanser & builder)

LOVE YOUR LIVER

Realizing the relevance of your bowel habits, it is important to restore balance to your glands for lasting weight management. Now is a good time to realize the part your liver plays to filter and clean the blood that has to oxygenate and feed the glands. Did you know that your liver is involved in as many as 200 crucial bodily functions? When you start RWR, I trust you will remember these words about your liver, and you will love your liver. Maybe it is time to put a picture of a heart on your bathroom mirror to remind yourself to love your liver. Help it and your colon each morning by drinking a warm cup of water with the juice of 1/2 a lemon or make Lemon Peel Tea (See page 105.) This will facilitate clearing the toxins that were filtered from the blood as you slept the night before.

Did you notice how drinking the herb teas or the warm lemonade helped to get things moving? Lemon juice, as well as some essential oils and herbs, help the liver to do its work for us. By drinking lemon juice water and teas we can help the liver purify the blood and produce bile.

Bile is a concentration of the toxins that the liver has filtered from the blood. Bile is released from the liver through the gallbladder into the large colon to excite the colon into peristalsis so we evacuate and cleanse the bowel. Bile also helps with the lysis or the break down of fats and cholesterol in the intestines. Do you see how the blood relies on this process? Again, Young Living's *Rehemogen Tincture* is the product I have used in my teas for liver, blood and colon cleansing when I have felt sluggish. Sluggishness usually means my liver needs a little more love. Dr. Bernard Jensen, PhD, taught for over sixty years and had thousands of case studies to show that the blood can only be clean when the liver and colon are clean.[20]

Some products specific to liver cleansing and health that I have taken over the years to help my body heal itself from liver and gallbladder congestion are the Young Living formulas of *JuvaTone, JuvaPower, JuvaSpice* supplements, and *JuvaCleanse*. Also *Release* and *JuvaFlex* essential oils blends and one bottle of *GLF,* a blend known to aid in eliminating the negative effects of toxins in the body as a gallbladder and liver cleanser. By this you can see that Young Living has quite a variety of products to help support our efforts to become and remain healthy. My gallbladder was removed 20 years ago so I have greatly appreciated these particular formulations.

I realize there are many things to remember if you've never eaten this way, and it does take some focus to do it. As you know, anything worthwhile will take some concentrated effort. For these four weeks of RWR, if I were you, I would be quite strict about sticking to the rules by eating all meals and snacks, and avoiding all items or activities known to delay or sabotage weight reduction like the toxic substances mentioned in the book and others found on the Environmental Working Group lists of toxic chemicals to avoid.[21]

It would be great if we could just talk about all the good things and ignore the negative aspects of the dietary and environmental challenges we face. Just think for a moment about how your body has an amazing ability to heal itself. Given a chance with cleansing and proper nutrition the liver can even regenerate, and we can have new blood cells every three months on our way back to a healthy weight.

In the segment on Kitchen Tools you'll find some tips that should make your path easier by organizing the kitchen for success. Not only will your liver love the healthy whole foods you prepare in your kitchen, your family and friends who eat there with you will too. At first, some members may not fully appreciate the changes you are making, but once you begin to model your new attitude, clarity of mind and slimmer body, any mumbles or grumbles you heard at the start will become words of admiration and appreciation for what you are accomplishing.

However, you may not be there yet, so if you didn't get around to reviewing the lists of foods and chemicals to avoid during the first week on the Environmental Working Group's lists then do so now. Your liver will love you as you avoid these irritants, and since certain negative emotions are thought to energetically affect the liver, your positive thoughts and happy emotions will be supporting its work, too.

CMS & RWR
Section 5: Table 3 - LEMON PEEL TEA

＊ Cleanse the rind of an organic, whole lemon with fruit & veggie wash.
＊ Cut into 4 quarters & put 2 in a mug.
＊ Cover with boiling water & steep for at least 10-20 minutes or longer.
＊ Do not add any sweetener.
＊ Drink warm either first thing in morning, before going to bed, or any time you feel the need to flush your system.

Lemon Peel Tea helps clear liver toxins & facilitates elimination.

WHAT YOU MAY EXPERIENCE

Are you choosing to try this lifestyle change to learn if it is for you? It makes sense, sounds healthy, and is evidently supported and promoted by many natural health advocates. You'll be feeling great in no time, right? Well, there's a good chance it won't happen as quickly as you'd like so please don't give up too soon.

Sugar, for example, is a tough one. You may have been avoiding it while flushing your body with plenty of drinking water and still it calls to you even after the withdrawal headaches are gone. We humans have emotional attachments to sweet foods, so our minds embrace them and we have to find ways to reeducate and distract our minds until we're free of the addiction (thought by some to be as difficult as giving up smoking or even cocaine). This is part of the reason CMS and RWR stresses how important it is to eat at least three protein meals each day, include healthy snacks, and become educated about the short-term and long-term benefits of being sugar-free.

Toxic substances have no doubt been building in your body for years, and you may endure certain symptoms of withdrawal once you discontinue ingesting them or eliminate exposure. If your health has deteriorated, it probably was not sudden. A weakened immune system can develop over a period of some time, and your digestive system might not have handled food in this pure form for ages. The good news though is that nature knows how to use fresh, whole foods, and if you have not degenerated far from your original design, then you will be able to recover digestive function. With patience and perseverance, you will see and FEEL the satisfying results of healthy living.

Some people experience a bit of discomfort like cravings, headaches, a faster heart rate, or even flu-like symptoms. These usually clear in about 3 to 7 days. If you realize this is just part of the process, then you won't sabotage reaching your weight goals or decide that eating this way is not worth the pain. Support the body systems experiencing distress with essential oils to clear the toxic residue. This way, you will not only feel much better quickly, you will also facilitate removal rather than covering pain symptoms or dulling them with pain pills, aspirin, ibuprofen, etc.

Young Living has many products that help with the stress of cleansing and digestive distress. *PanAway* is a pain formula that can banish a headache almost instantly when a drop is gently massaged into the temples and at the hairline along the back of the neck. *Stress Away Roll-On* is very helpful throughout the process of eliminating sugars and starches. The luscious fragrance may help lessen the desire to overeat along with stress release. *Peace & Calming* is a favorite for nervous tension, helps with restful sleep, and calms restless legs. Diffusing into your work and home environment will be a beneficial habit to cultivate. Try *Purification, Sacred Frankincense* and/or *Clarity.*

Dr. Stanley Bass, ND, DC, explained, the body's natural processes when cleansing, saying: "When quality natural foods are introduced, remarkable things begin to happen to the body as well as the mind. The amazing intelligence present in every cell of your body and the wisdom of the body immediately manifests itself. The rule may be stated that when the quality of food coming into the body is of higher quality than the tissues that the body is made of, the body begins to discard the lower-grade materials and tissues. It makes room for the superior materials that it uses to make new and healthier tissue. This is the plan of nature. The body is very selective and ALWAYS aims for improvement and better health. The body always tries to produce health and always will, unless our interference is too great."[22]

CMS & RWR
Section 5: Table 4
DRY SKIN BRUSHING

With a natural bristle brush, start at the feet brushing in circular fashion up one leg then the other, up the thighs, buttocks, moving upward, then do the arms and gently across the chest and down the back.

✳ Dry skin brushing facilitates the release of toxins, helps lymph flow, circulation and exfoliates dead skin cells.

✳ Use skin creams and lotions sparingly. Products applied to our skin must be metabolized through the liver and broken down like fats without first being processed by digestive enzymes.

✳ Use personal products formulated with all natural ingredients. Products applied to our skin and head such as toothpastes, mouthwashes, lipsticks, shampoos, conditioners, etc. do not get digested through enzyme action like injested foods. Chemical toxins in personal care products burden body tissues like our glands and lymph system, and are held in fat cells until cleansed when and if the body is able to do so.

✳ Dry skin brushing will especially benefit those who do not perspire regularly.

STRESS AND WEIGHT REDUCTION

Have you noticed an underlying theme of how body chemistry is created and performs according to the quality of our thoughts, the foods we eat and environment? Because you are serious about weight reduction, you will want to understand how both internal and external stress negatively affect your efforts, and how stress can be relieved naturally.

Physiological stress is "a specific response by the body to a stimulus, as a fear or pain, that disturbs or interferes with the normal physiological equilibrium of an organism."[23] When you feel anxious, pressured, burdened or worried, these emotional states disturb your normal chemistry or internal equilibrium. Your body is equipped to deal with stress, because we all experience it from time to time, but when stress is a constant state of being then you must become aware and choose to change the patterns that cause you to be so stressed.

If you deem your stress levels manageable by yourself, then some of the helpful tips given in this Section will benefit you. As we have already learned, stress is messing with the endocrine messengers like neuropeptide Y from the hypothalamus. If changing your diet to the CMS plan produces more stress than you can overcome, then it will be counterproductive. To succeed at your weight reduction goals, a personal consultant may be able to help you with stress reduction.

Also, there are holistic practitioners who are able to coach us through our challenges from the viewpoint of wholeness; spirit, mind and body. Some helpers who work specifically with stress release are Massage Therapists, Yoga Teachers, Ti Chi Teachers, and Emotional Release Technique

Practitioners who use tapping or specific therapeutic-grade essential oils. Modalities that are often holistic and help with relieving stress are Aromatherapy, Chiropractic treatments, Flower Remedies, Homeopathy, Hydrotherapy, Hypnosis, Naturopathy, Reiki and, of course, Nutritionists, among others. Professional Health Coaches can also be helpful.

The National Library of Medicine and the National Institutes of Health at Medline Plus[24] have online services that teach about stress and identify its causes. Being aware of the clues and cues in and around you will help you know how to continue. The American Psychological Association website is another resource warning, "Stress that is left unchecked or poorly managed is known to contribute to high blood pressure, heart disease, obesity, diabetes..."[25] In their list of warning signals the body sends to alert that extra care is needed are diet and eating related signs such as a lack of appetite or increased appetite for "comfort foods or other digestive upsets."[26]

Stress from external sources that exert undue burden on you should be considered, too. Among these are relationships, home and work environments, excessive temperature variations or noise, finances, and/or illness of yourself or a close loved one. We each must find our way through our individual challenges. Fortunately, the human systems are quite resourceful and resilient. If your resilience is worn a bit too thin due to the stress of your circumstances, it may be time to seek support from spiritual or professional services.

When we work or play into the night after the earth signals "lights out" at sundown, then we interrupt important phases of our sleep and restoration cycles. Exposing yourself to flickering lights late at night by watching television or playing electronic games will cause the head glands to produce the chemicals that keep us alert, and throw off the timing of restoration orchestrated by those glands. Try having lights out by 10 to 10:30 p.m. to allow your body to reorient itself to nature's flow. Healing energies ebb and flow according to the natural sun cycles and time zones in which we live. Sleep in total darkness to give the head glands the rest they need from the alert state before they begin to direct the body's healing and cleansing activities during sleep. Remove all glowing light sources from your sleeping room or cover them if they must remain. Do not use a night light in your room or in a baby's or child's room. Night lights can be installed in a hallway and a flashlight is handy if you need to be up in the night.

Lack of sleep is a stress that can be a problem for overweight and obese people. Another Medline Plus article out of the National Library of Medicine and the American Journal of Clinical Nutrition claims that, "People eat more when they are starved for sleep." The interesting theory researched by Dr. Laurent Brondel and Dr. Damien Davenne of France postulates, "It's possible that people might eat more after a short sleep because mammals have evolved to store up calories in the summer, when nights are short and food is plentiful."[27] They confirm and expand on my conclusions about repair and recovery by stating, "It is time to understand that sleep is not just losing time, besides the recovery processes that occur, there are many other functions (energy conservation, memory, and so on) which are going on."[28]

If lack of sleep is an area of stress for you, know that many people have found relief once they introduced therapeutic-grade essential oils into their lives. Applying oils that have calming and relaxing properties such as *Lavender* and citrus oils like *Orange* or the blend *Citrus Fresh* soothe and assist with this. Diffusing specific essential oils in the room as you sleep is another way to ensure rest. *RutaVaLa Roll-On* or *Stress Away Roll-On* from Young Living are perfect to help with sleep, as well as their encapsulated essential oils supplement, *SleepEssence*. A favorite at our house is the supplement with melatonin, *ImmuPro*. The best help yet for me and other menopausal women with whom I've spoken who had previously lacked quality sleep due to hormone imbalances has been Young Living's product released at the 2010 Annual Convention, *Progessence Plus Serum*. Just giving our bodies a few drops of this serum by applying it over the carotid area on our necks has been very effective for better, deeper rest.

It may be that an acidic pH is causing restlessness and a lack of quality sleep. Maintaing the pH of the blood is a very high priority for the body to constantly perform. If we do not supply through diet or supplementation the mineral ions needed to maintain equilibrium of this crucial chemistry, minerals will be drawn away from other tissues as long as the body can do so. The nervous system, bones, teeth and other tissues can give up minerals they need because the blood must remain slightly alkaline at 7.35 to 7.4 pH. The acidic person is restless and sometimes feels antsy. Do you think a diet rich in colorful fruits, vegetables and seeds could help provide the needed minerals? There are also several Young Living vitamin and mineral supplements from which to choose such as *Alkalime, MultiGreens, Master*

Formula Hers/His, True Source, SuperCal, MegaCal, Mineral Essence, Super C, Super B and *NingXia Red* antioxidant juice infusion.

Therapeutic-grade essential oils will digest acids, thereby assisting in raising the body's pH. This is one very valuable benefit to help us deal with the major stress of being too acidic. Consistency is key, but it works in such a pleasing and easy way. The oils do work! When a person remarks that an essential oil single or blend "does nothing for me," I often suspect if it were a pure, therapeutic-grade that the chemistry of the oils did help to bring up their pH even temporarily. It can be that the regulation of blood pH was a higher priority than relieving discomfort or some other reason for using the essential oil.

Stress also draws on our stores of the element chlorine. When we eat protein, the stomach must produce hydrochloric acid (HCL) as one of the digestive chemical compounds that begins to break down protein foods for absorption. The amount of hydrogen available in this process is dependent on how much chlorine is present to create the needed HCL for the stomach to release at the time of digestion. If stress has depleted the supply of chlorine then we will have insufficient HCL with incomplete digestion results. Has a meal ever felt like a rock or big lump in your stomach? That's a body cue that it's time to kick back, de-stress, and maybe eat some digestive enzymes. So it is with a hyperacid stomach condition that can be felt as acid reflux. Don't be deceived by the TV ads promising relief from excess stomach acid by taking antacids. They may relieve the burning temporarily, but this will not correct the origins of the problem of digestive insufficiency.

Diet, exercise and avoiding toxic substances to the best of our abilities are powerful influences that we can control to support how our bodies will react to stress. The following list has some ideas you may also choose to adopt:

★ Do deep breathing exercises, especially when anxious, panicked or feeling too acidic. (Maybe being acidic exacerbates anxious feelings?)

★ Take a warm bath with high quality, therapeutic-grade essential oils infused in a bath gel base.

★ Talk to an understanding friend.

★ Apply Young Living's *Stress Away Roll-On, RutaVaLa Roll-On, Tranquil Roll-On, Peace & Calming* blend, *Sacred Frankincense,* and/or *Lavender.*

★ Play music or soothing nature sounds.

★ Draw and/or paint a picture.

★ Practice forgiveness. "Let not the sun go down on your wrath."[29]

★ Use sound frequency technology specifically designed to entrain the brainwaves for deep relaxation.

★ Meditate or sit in listening prayer.

★ Take a walk in the fresh air and sunshine.

★ Allow the sun to warm your shoulders.

★ Work in a flower or vegetable garden. Watch birds.

★ Laugh and be playful. Remember being childlike; watch children play.

★ Join a team just for fun - with only healthy competition.

★ Volunteer for charity or help a neighbor.

★ Dance if it causes you to feel good.

★ Read an uplifting book.

★ Have an Aromatherapy massage or foot rub.

★ Learn self-hypnosis.

★ Have a manicure and/or pedicure and relax.

★ Associate with others who appreciate and support your new lifestyle.

★ Communicate with others, "sweet people,"who are kicking the sugars habit.

★ Use Internet tools to find helps and supportive products.

CMS & RWR
Section 5: Table 5 - DID YOU KNOW

...that 1 cup of coffee or 1 alcoholic beverage requires many glasses of water to recover from the dehydration that results?

...that coffee and alcohol leech essential vitamins & minerals?

...that water transports oxygen to your cells, helps you digest & absorb nutrients, & gets rid of toxins & solid wastes?

...that drinking water lubricates your joints & keeps your skin moist?

...that drinking Green tea may assist with reducing weight.

...that *Ocotea* is an essential oil from Ecuador that may increase a feeling of fullness* that may be diffused, inhaled, diluted for topical application or used as a dietary supplement. *Ocotea* is also found in the luscious blend, *Stress Away Roll-On*.

This statement has not been evaluated by the Food & Drug Administration.

EXERCISE

As you can see, I have delayed the subject of exercise until you are well into the book so I didn't scare you away at first glance. This is one area that is absolutely scientifically proven to be one of the best, if not THE best, for relieving stress, giving our glands and organs a natural massage, and helps to increase metabolism through increased muscle mass. Because it has been a struggle between what I know to do for myself in this area and then not doing it, I have found a few helpful ways to get my body moving even when I don't feel like it.

Some joys of life are that the human body is designed to move and breathe. Since most of us are not out hunting or walking in the woods to gather in our meals, the exercise experts have developed all sorts of programs for us. That's why I'm not going to even pretend that I can advise anything about exercise except to say that you and I both know we need to be moving, moving, moving. This also means strength training that strengthens the muscles with the advantage of then strengthening the bones. How important do you think having strong bones will be to our goals of longevity?

I have come to understand that effective cardio work can be accomplished in 20 minutes just two times a week. Dr. Joseph Mercola explains how and why the "PEAK" type of cardio is so beneficial and how it can help to increase Human Growth Hormone (HGH). You may visit his web site to read the complete article (See Bibliography.), but here are the benefits he listed:[30]

- Lowers your body fat
- Dramatically improves muscle tone
- Firms your skin and reduces wrinkles
- Boosts your energy and sexual desire
- Improves athletic speed and performance
- Allows you to achieve your fitness goals much faster

The above list could have been describing results of achieving hormone balance in our bodies. Exercise is one component of over-all health that helps to enhance hormone production - especially for blood sugar regulation and Human Growth Hormone. HGH begins to wane as we reach our 30's. Young Living developed an oral spray of essential oils and other nutrients that supports pituitary gland function to enhance HGH production. Spraying *Ultra Young Plus Oral Spray* inside the cheeks twice daily is thought to help increase this important hormone which is most compatible with CMS and RWR because we have eliminated eating sugars. Also, Dr. Mercola explains in the above mentioned article why drinking sports drinks soon after workouts is counterproductive:

"If you consume sugar or fructose, especially within two hours post-exercise, you will increase somatostatin which will in turn obliterate the production of growth hormone! This is yet another example of why gulping down sports drinks that are chockfull of high fructose corn syrup can do your body more harm than good, and will just shut down your body's production of HGH and negate many of the benefits from your exercise."[31]

It is best to eat protein after working out to help with muscle recovery. This is an ideal time to drink a smoothie with any of Young Living's protein powders of *Pure Protein Complete, Power Meal* or *Balance Complete*. Also, some exercise keys are:

★ Wear a pedometer and increase the number of steps you take each week.

★ Use a mini-trampoline or rebounder to do the health bounce, jog or dance.

★ Use hand weights to strengthen bones, joints and tone arms while walking outside or treadmill or doing the health-bounce on a mini-trampoline rebounder.

★ Using weights may trick your body into thinking it must step up the metabolism due to the extra exertion required by the added weight "burden."

★ Use Vibration Plates equipment. (Reasonably priced and do not require much room. My favorite if I don't feel like exercising or if time is limited.)

★ Use an undulating perpetual motion machine like the Chi Machine.

★ Walk with a friend or walk a dog friend.

Section 6

"Your kitchen is
the Laboratory of Life,
YOU are the chemist...
Be sure you know your business!"

~ Dr. Hazel R. Parcells, PhD, DC, ND
Nutritional Advisor

KITCHEN HELPS

I love kitchen gadgets, but I have found a few that are more useful than others to make food prep go smoothly. Besides the usual collection of pots and pans, a set of sharp knives is a good investment. I especially like to use a long bread knife for sectioning citrus fruits. Some additional, indispensable kitchen tools are:

+ a mandolin for fine slicing

+ a hand-operated chopper

+ cutting boards that can be thoroughly cleansed

+ a steamer and a tea kettle

+ a smoothie maker - to grind nuts and seeds, too

+ a little food processor

+ green storage bags that extend freshness

+ a food scale

+ a colander and/or strainer/drainer

+ some food storage bins - used glass jars with lids work great

+ a handy little counter top grill that allows for oils and fats to drain easily

+ a quality juicer

+ *Thieves Household Cleaner* and *Thieves Wipes*

+ *Diffuser, Lemon* essential oil and *Purification* essential oil

+ a question mark (?) sign on the refrigerator door to reinforce your WHY

Creating healthy kitchen chemistry depends on the time and effort you have to invest. Most of us need to find efficient ways and tools to get it all done. The above items are self explanatory, but I like to promote the use of those green storage bags. Prepare batches of chopped veggies to have ready to simply pull from the refrigerator to make a quick and colorful salad or sauteed meal. I separate the vegetable categories in these bags. Green leafy veggies are combined in one or diced peppers of several colors in another.

Though once cut, fruits and vegetables begin to oxidize and lose valuable vitamins and enzymes, these green bags help to slow the process during storage. It is best to eat plant foods soon after preparing them, but if convenience is called for, a good, quick meal is created in minutes by having some of the basic color categories ready to use.

Of course, the trick is to have cleaned and prepared the veggies soon after bringing them in from the market or garden. Since we are avoiding chemical pesticides, I make a "green" cleansing solution of water with Young Living's *Thieves Household Cleaner* and a few drops of *Lemon* essential oil. All of our fruits, vegetables and greens receive this bath, are rinsed well in clear water then drained or spun dried before being separated into their green bags. Practically everything in the refrigerator goes into these handy bags to extend the life and freshness of the produce, and to prevent any flavors or fragrances from blending.

Tip: Keep a spray bottle handy with the *Thieves Household Cleaner* and *Lemon* essential oil when you only have a few items to cleanse of agricultural chemicals, waxes, etc. You can also spray with white or apple cider vinegar and follow with 3% hydrogen peroxide (from the drugstore) then rinse well, but be careful the peroxide doesn't bleach linens.

The Young Living *Thieves* product line is wonderful for eliminating kitchen smudges and food related bacteria. Several essential oils, especially the citrus oils like *Lemon* and *Orange,* can leave the room totally refreshed without adding harmful chemicals. A few drops of *Lemon* essential oil mixed into a tablespoon of olive oil can be used to polish wood cabinets which also leaves a true lemon-fresh scent and provides healthy, non toxic exercise. (Always test a spot to be sure the materials are compatible.) *Purification* is another blend very useful to diffuse as its name implies.

Since essential oils are very concentrated, the rule is to be cautious and conservative when getting started with physical applications and around fabrics and furniture. Never allow a bottle of essential oils to sit on a painted surface. The solvent properties of the oils can dissolve petrol-based chemical compounds. You can see it work if you perform a simple test by putting water in a Styrofoam cup with a drop or two of *Lemon* essential oil. Allow it to sit for a few minutes. The oils will literally dismantle the Styrofoam at the water line. This is a good visual for you to realize how the essential oils are capable of cleaning receptor sites from any petroleum-based film that could be hindering cellular function. This is a good thing.

A note about plastics in the kitchen: Any plastic container that gives up its shape in the dishwasher is not a safe plastic for food storage. Also, DO NOT microwave foods in any plastic containers. The chemicals used to produce this plastic break down when microwaved and can be detrimental to health. We now have generations of people who have been exposed to these chemicals through microwaving plastics. Who knows what the cumulative effects have been on human DNA? Questions arise about the properties of plastic bottles and containers being linked to levels of toxins known to be carcinogenic or to disrupt hypothalamus function. The developing brains and nervous systems of infants and young children are especially vulnerable.

YOUNG LIVING ESSENTIAL OILS
SECTION 6: TABLE 1 - KITCHEN HELPS

Diffusers
Lavender Foaming Hand Soap
Lavender Hand & Body Lotion
LavaDerm Cooling Mist
Lemon & Orange essential oils
Purification essential oil blend
Thieves essential oil blend
Thieves Foaming Hand Soap
Thieves Concentrated Houshold Cleaner
Thieves Wipes
Young Living Cookbook, Volume 1
Healthy Cooking for body, mind, & soul
A variety of YLTG™ essential oils

CONVERTING RECIPES

Practically every favorite meal or recipe can be creatively converted to accommodate CMS and RWR. The only difference is the limited or eliminated ingredients that fall under the RWR plan because of their higher caloric or lower nutritional values. Most recipes don't need all the sugars and fats they usually call for. A little "Better Butter" goes a long way for flavoring and moistness, and a little unsweetened apple sauce or fresh fruit juices like pineapple or orange do quite nicely for sweetening when on CMS. Use stevia (sweet leaf) for sweetening for CMS and especially when on RWR. It has a Glycemic Index of zero.

Here's a short list of dishes I've been able to convert from old favorites to give you some idea. I simply add to the traditional ingredients to include most of the food categories called for by CMS and RWR:

+ Mexican recipes like enchiladas, burritos, tacos, tostadas, etc.

+ Italian recipes including salads and other Mediterranean-type dishes.

+ Meatloaf: I grind green cabbage or grate zucchini as the "filler" instead of using oatmeal or cereal flakes that some recipes call for.

+ I use chopped parsley in almost everything; even in green onion, and cottage cheese pancakes.

+ In Indian recipes I go easy on the potatoes, but love the spices.

+ Thai recipes made with coconut milk, curry and all the veggie groups go well over long grain brown rice.

✦ With Chinese menus I can use all the crunchy veggies and control the fat content by fixing them at home. Long grain brown rice is preferred.

✦ Traditional salads, like Caesar and Waldorf, are expanded by adding other items to complete the colored categories and making adjustments to the dressings with healthy oils.

✦ The easiest of all is a beautiful array of the veggie categories presented attractively on a platter for raw grazing.

✦ Overnight guests are greeted with a fruit-grazing tray of beautiful and juicy appetizers of freshly cut fruits (kiwi, blueberries, oranges, strawberries, raspberries, apricots, prunes, grapes and banana chunks) and *wolfberries* with nuts that have been soaked overnight such as raw cashews, walnuts, almonds, and pumpkin seeds. This tray, with a cup of herb tea, satisfies the early risers very nicely.

EATING OUT OR ON THE ROAD

You probably aren't going to find a sign posted in plain sight on the fence or door of your neighborhood restaurant declaring DANGER! BEWARE OF SUGAR. (Unless they have a guard dog named Sugar.) You must enter cautiously, armed with knowledge. Of course there are several other hazards lurking in most modern eateries too, like high sodium, hydrogenated and rancid fats, over-processed bleached flours, etc. However, there are some choices that you will find palatable and consistent with your diet.

It is best if you can help it, to not be too hungry or too tired when you enter restaurants. Being mindful of your circumstance you must prepare for delays and possibly a menu that doesn't support your new way of eating. The menu could also show pictures of meals you used to eat that can stimulate cravings - especially if you are hungry or experiencing a drop in blood sugar. Try to have in mind what you are going to order ahead of time so you don't have to give much time and energy to reviewing the menu. Look for preparation methods that you use at home like baked, grilled, steamed or broiled. A fresh salad bar should have all the food categories presented so choose something from each color to enjoy a well balanced salad.

Most restaurants have a fresh "house salad" that can be your first line of defense when ordering in these dangerous environments. Tell your waitperson that you are on a special diet and must avoid sodium, sugar and fats. Ask for specifics about what is in the house salad, and ask for dressings on the side. Also, from now on, ask for extra lemon wedges to squeeze the juice on everything. Perhaps instead of salad dressing you could carry your own.

You may need to order from the a la carte' portion of the menu to find smaller serving sizes or when practicing proper food combining. Choose a lean protein to eat after the salad OR a yam or boiled potato. Eating out will probably tax your digestive functions so it's best to refrain from eating proteins and starches at the same meal. Realize that if you want a slice of the bread or a roll, and you will be ordering a baked potato or yam to eat with the salad, these two items will fulfill your starch requirements for the whole day. If you've already had one starch for the day, then salad with a meat serving is a better choice unless you are willing to eat only the potato or the bread, but not both.

Prepare and carry a 3x5 card with you that lists the foods you have chosen to restrict. Having this handy when you are ordering will impress upon the server how important this is to you, and he or she will usually become your ally in asking the kitchen to fulfill your dietary needs. The card helps you to remember to ask about things like if the potatoes are soaked in salt water before baking, what oils are used, or if the fish is wild caught or farm raised.

As mentioned in the Portions or Servings segment, there's a good chance that you will be served enough food for two meals. Eat all the salad with one-half of the protein and take the rest home. Ask for your take-home box to be brought out with your food so you can divide it before you begin to eat. If you leave this to the end of the meal, you will find that most of the time you will eat more than intended. Some kitchens will divide your meal for you before serving it. If the note is written on your 3x5 card, again the waitperson will see how important it is to you and will help ease your eating out challenge.

Some ethnic restaurants such as Chinese, Japanese, Thai and Indian tend to serve dishes with plenty of colorful, fresh vegetables, and their meat and fish portions are generally smaller, but skip the rice and noodles. Italian restaurants usually serve chicken, meat and seafood dishes that can be ordered without pasta, and you can request vegetable side dishes prepared without "extra" salt and olive oil.

The key to eating out is to mindfully prepare beforehand, then afterwards expect to drink some parsley tea or Lemon Peel Tea to help with flushing any excess sodium. Also, make sure you carry food digestive enzymes with you to take with the meal.

Prepare the best you can when invited to eat meals hosted by friends and family. Good fellowship is essential, and meal time makes for gracious social time. Eat what you can then leave what you can without offending anyone. Allow your friends and family to know your weight reduction plans as you solicit their support.

TRIPS BY ROAD & BY AIR

A road trip does require planning. It's a good idea to take along digestive enzymes and bottles of *Peppermint* and *Di-Gize* essential oils.

+ Plan to eat a hearty breakfast each day then eat lightly the rest of the day. Plan snacks to gradually maintain blood sugar the duration of the trip.

+ Before leaving home, do a web search for restaurants located along the projected route. Many restaurants post their menus on their web sites. Decide where you plan to eat meals before you leave home.

+ Carry two coolers in the car that fit behind the front seats or will be easy to reach. Fill one with a supply of your own water, and the second with tubs or sacks of finger-food snacks of sliced peppers, cucumbers, baby carrots, grape tomatoes and tri-colored peppers. Carry walnuts and soaked almonds for brain food protein snacks.

+ When carrying essential oils with you, provide a cool spot for them, and do not leave them in a closed car where the heat will rise.

+ Oranges make refreshing, stress-reducing roadside snacks when taking a rest break. Other fruits, like apples, that are not so juicy, can be munched safely along the way.

+ Carry tea bags and individual hot cups. When you stop for a rest break and to gas up, fill your personal cups with hot water from the coffee station at the gas station.

+ Carry Young Living's *NingXia Red* juice packets (1 oz) in the cooler for a quick energy pick up. It is a concentrated antioxidant infusion.

+ When flying, request a Vegan meal if provided, but carry snacks like soaked almonds, apples or oranges and stay hydrated with water.

Depending upon your mode of transportation, the above eating out tips apply to when you travel too.

YOUNG LIVING ESSENTIAL OILS

Section 6: Table 2 - TRIPS BY ROAD OR AIR

- *NingXia Red* 1 ounce sample packets are perfect to take along when traveling.
- Drink *NingXia Red* as you go along for sustained energy & immune support.
- *Thieves Spray & Thieves Wipes* protect from germs in public restrooms.
- Use *Thieves Waterless Hand Sanitizer* after using public restrooms, touching hand rails and straps, escalators, & shopping carts.
- *Thieves Lozenges* are convenient to help keep sinuses and head clear.
- *Peppermint* essential oil soothes the digestion, boosts energy & is cooling.
- Tip: Keep a handkerchief or cloth damp & cool in your travel cooler. Put *Peppermint* on the back of your neck then rest the damp cloth on the neck to help with fatigue & hot weather driving or anytime when heat is uncomfortable.
- *Rosemary* essential oil helps to keep drivers alert. Place a drop or two on a paper blotter or piece of felt cloth. Locate it on the dashboard where the sun hits it. Move the paper as the direction of the sun shifts. This is called the "Truckers Oil."
- **NOTE:** Protect plastic materials when using essential oils.

RECIPES FROM RITA'S KITCHEN

SIMPLE SALAD DRESSING

2 tsp olive oil

1 TBS apple cider vinegar or fresh squeezed lemon juice

A pinch or two of unrefined sea salt (optional)

1/2 tsp to 1 tsp of fresh or dried herbs of choice

Whisk all together and pour over salad contents.

SIMPLE CMS SALAD FOR ONE

1 C cut Romaine lettuce (or other lettuce of choice - preferably not iceberg lettuce)

1/2 C finely sliced cucumber - about 1/2 medium cucumber

2-3 green onions sliced

1/4 green bell pepper diced or sliced

1/4 red bell pepper (or tomato) diced or sliced

1/4 C finely cut parsley

2 sliced red radishes

Toss with Simple Salad Dressing

Note: May add cold turkey or chicken or 1 hard boiled egg.

Toppings: thinly sliced or shredded purple cabbage and/or carrot, fresh ground flax seeds or 2 TBS sprouted alfalfa, chia, sunflower or pumpkin seeds

CUCUMBER NON-FAT DRESSING

1 organic cucumber, washed and sliced

1 clove of garlic, chopped or pressed

Italian dry herb seasoning to taste OR dill weed.

Blend all ingredients until liquid, adjust taste and refrigerate.

Use on any salad or the dill dressing with fish.

May add apple cider vinegar, especially if eating red meat.

Note: This is your take-along dressing since there is no oil to go rancid. Carry some with you when you go out to eat. It combines well with any foods found on a menu except fruit.

CINNAMON TOAST

1 slice organic rye bread (or 50 cal toast of choice)

Blend 1 tsp organic coconut oil with 1/4 to 1/2 tsp ground cinnamon.

The sweet leaf supplement, *stevia*, mixes well in combination with cinnamon.

While bread is toasting, blend coconut oil, cinnamon and stevia with a spatula or flat knife on a plate. Immediately spread this mixture on toasted bread while hot.

Note: Organic coconut oil is good for us, up to 2 TBS per day on CMS. (RWR restrict to 1 to 2 tsp a day.) Cinnamon helps regulate blood sugar.

SPINACH OMELET FOR ONE

1 fresh egg whisked w/1/4 tsp water. (may add extra egg white)

1 to 2 C spinach, washed, steamed separately for 3 minutes without adding water.

A sprinkle of unrefined sea salt (optional)

1 TBS organic apple cider vinegar

1 TBS chopped green onion and/or garlic

1 TBS snipped parsley & 1 tsp chia seeds

Heat omelet pan and spray with very little olive oil or use a bit of coconut oil. Pour whisked egg & water into pan to cook.

Put vinegar, green onion and garlic in spinach and stir.

When ready, place cooked egg on plate then put the drained, steamed spinach mixture on 1/2 the circle then fold the other 1/2 over like a taco. Sprinkle parsley and chia seeds over the top. Serve with tomato slices, bell pepper strips and jicama or radish.

BAKED ZUCCHINI

1 large zucchini sliced in half lengthwise, scoop out pulp

3-4 green onions

1 stalk of celery with some celery tops

1 TBS curly parsley

1 egg whisked

1/4 tsp dry basil or 3 medium sized fresh basil leaves

In food processor blend pulp, onion, celery, egg, basil & parsley.

Place zucchini shells in baking dish with about 1/4 inch of water in the bottom and fill shells with mixture.

Bake in 350° oven for 30 minutes.

PARSLEY OR WOLFBERRY PANCAKES - 2 versions

1/2 C low fat, organic cottage cheese or ricotta cheese

1 egg

3 TBS gluten-free flour or pancake mix

1/4 C parsley OR 1/4 C dried *NingXia Wolfberries*

4 green onions chopped (in parsley pancakes, not in wolfberry pancakes)

Blend all ingredients in smoothie maker, blender or food processor.

Pour on hot griddle and cook until brown and the steam mostly stops.

Note: If eaten with 1 tsp of Better Butter, this recipe will count for a protein, a fat (a fruit if wolfberry), and a starch serving for the day.

Hint: Make colorful fresh salsa or pico to eat with the parsley pancakes.

SPINACH OR KALE SAUTE'

1 bunch of greens

1 tsp organic coconut oil

Sprinkling of garlic powder

4 to 5 green onions

1 TBS organic apple cider vinegar

Wash and rinse spinach, kale or greens

In heavy pot saute' sliced green onions in coconut oil.

Gently steam greens in pot with onions and vinegar. Sprinkle with garlic powder to taste.

BRAISED ASPARAGUS

Lightly spray large frying pan with olive oil or coat with coconut oil. Arrange washed asparagus (leave some water on it) single layer in the pan. Sprinkle with grains of sea salt, and dry herb mix. Cook asparagus al dente a few minutes, stir lightly so they don't stick.

KEFIR CHEESE OR GREEK YOGURT CHEESE

CMS allows for about 1 ounce of hard cheeses every few days, but it is always best to avoid the soft, creamy cheese preparations. RWR participants should forego all cheese, but may make a respectable, friendly bacteria yogurt or Kefir cheese as substitute for cream cheese if absolutely a necessity.

Pour plain liquid Kefir (no sweetener or fruit) into cheesecloth stretched over a bowl or into a cheese funnel. Drain overnight.

Cover to retain freshness, then refrigerate. (Use drained liquid in a smoothie.)

Use Kefir cheese instead of sour cream or cream cheese. (RWR limit.)

Note: Kefir cheese will be thinner in texture, and has a mild taste. For a thicker "cheese" drain nonfat or low-fat Greek yogurt. Add a little stevia to Greek Yogurt Cheese and serve with 1/4 C blueberries. (Try different brands of stevia to find the taste you like the best.)

AVOCADO DRESSING OR GUACAMOLE

1 avocado, peeled and pitted

1/2 to 1 small to medium sized organic cucumber washed and sliced

1 clove of garlic chopped or pressed

1/2 lime juiced

Blend all ingredients starting with only 1/2 of cucumber so mixture stays rather thick, adjust taste and refrigerate. Use as salad dressing.(RWR limit to 1 TBS.) Serve as guacamole with Jicama spears for appetizer.

BAKED ACORN SQUASH

(1/4 C is 1 of 3 for week's starch servings.)

1 acorn squash cut in half with seeds cleaned out

1 tsp Better Butter (See recipe.)or organic coconut oil

1/2 tsp ground cinnamon

1/4 to 1/2 tsp ground nutmeg

Dry split acorn squash with paper towel, & rub cut surfaces with 1 tsp Better Butter or coconut oil

Mix spices and sprinkle over and inside of squash

Bake at 400° for about an hour.

Serve with steamed cauliflower. Good with fresh ground turkey meat loaf.

Serve with salad of mixed leafy greens.

COLOR ME SLIM TURKEY MEATLOAF

Olive oil spray or coconut oil (enough to coat pan)

2 lbs fresh ground turkey

1/2 cup ground or shredded cabbage or zuchinni for fiber and moisture

2 large eggs

1 medium onion finely chopped

1/4 C finely snipped parsley

1 tsp dried oregano and/or 1 tsp dried thyme or use fresh or dried sage

1/2 tsp unrefined sea salt

1/4 tsp pepper

1 clove of garlic finely chopped (optional)

3/4 cup gluten free bread crumbs made from rice or sprouted grain bread (RWR & CI omit, and add more shredded cabbage.)

Preheat oven to 400 degrees F. Coat an 11 by 9 inch baking dish with olive oil spray or coconut oil. In a large bowl, lightly beat the eggs. Add the oregano, thyme, salt, pepper; stir. Add the turkey, cabbage, parsley and bread crumbs; mix until combined. Transfer the mixture to the baking dish, and form into a loaf. Bake until a meat thermometer inserted into the thickest part of the loaf registers 165 degrees F, about 45 minutes. Let stand for 5 minutes before serving.

RICE, AMARANTH OR QUINOA PILAF

(1/4 C is 1 of 3 for the week's starch servings).

1 C of organic long grain brown rice, amaranth or quinoa (rinsed)

2 C of water brought to a boil

4-5 green onions minced

1/2 C red pepper chopped small

1/2 C parsley

1 clove garlic

1/2 carrot chopped small

Rinse rice, amaranth or quinoa well. Slowly pour uncooked grains into boiling water, stir until water returns to a boil so grain does not stick.

Note: organic chicken broth may be used instead of water, but only bring it to a slow boil before adding the grains.

Stir in all vegetables, reduce heat to a simmer until the water is absorbed.

Serve with any non-starch vegetables or green salad.

COLOR ME SLIM STUFFED BELL PEPPERS

1 or 2 green bell peppers with tops cut off, cored and cleaned

1 C cooked brown rice or quinoa pilaf (or fresh corn if not on RWR)

1 onion chopped

1/2 red pepper or pimento pepper diced

1/2 C green beans cooked and cut diagonally

1 tsp - 1 TBS Italian herb mix or favorite herb mix

Mix all ingredients and stuff green bell pepper shells.

Bake in covered casserole, 400° for 30 minutes.

COLOR ME SLIM STUFFED TOMATOES

2 to 4 tomatoes cleaned and cored

1 can albacore tuna (packed in water) or 1 C organic, low-fat cottage cheese

4 green onions chopped

1 to 2 celery stalks with leaves chopped

1 to 2 TBS parsley snipped or chopped

Garlic powder (optional)

2 TBS Cucumber-Dill Salad Dressing

Drain tuna, mix with veggies (add dressing if too dry), stuff tomatoes.

Serve with sprouted sunflower or pumpkin seeds.

Serve on a bed of lettuce or spinach leaves with cucumber dressing with raw snap peas, baby carrot and rye crackers.

ALMOND-DATE BALLS

(CMS very limited, RWR restricted, CI totally restricted!)

In food processor combine 1/2 C soaked organic almonds, & 1/2 C pitted dates. Process till the nuts & dates are chopped into medium size pieces. Add 1 small, peeled & seeded orange & mix. (Optional: Dip a toothpick in *Orange* essential oil then drag it back and forth through the mixture.) Make balls of 1 tsp of mix & roll in fresh coconut (optional). High sugar, beware!

BETTER BUTTER

(CI restricted due to milk sugar.)

Allow 1/2 C (1 stick) of unsalted, <u>organic</u> butter come to room temperature then blend with 1/2 C of organic virgin olive oil, 1/8 to 1/4 tsp of unrefined sea salt (optional) and 1 TBS <u>non-GMO</u> lecithin granules until well mixed. Transfer to nonporous or glass jar and refrigerate.

Hint: make this mix in a food processor then, instead of washing out the residue, chop some onion, garlic, parsley and oregano or other herbs to saute for an Italian dish.

Note: Use ONLY organic butter. The high fat of cream can hold any agricultural chemicals use in commercially raised cows in the fat molecules thus being concentrated in commercial butter.

SESAME SEED WAFFLES

(CI and RWR restricted)

Combine 1 cup of water with 1 cup of sesame seeds in the blender. Blend, then add 1 more cup of water. Blend again, then use the mixture in place of liquid in gluten-free Pancake/Waffle Mix. Add 2 eggs and 1 tablespoon of coconut oil. Bake on hot waffle iron until light brown. Serve with Young Living's *Blue Agave* nectar or make a syrup by gently heating 1/4 cup *Blue Agave* nectar, 1 sliced banana, 1 tablespoon of coconut oil and 1/4 cup walnut pieces. Serve warm.

PARSLEY TEA

1 C of packed down organic parsley (curly leaf) or 1 TBS dry parsley

Place parsley in glass, Pyrex or stainless steel bowl.

Cover parsley with 1 quart of boiling water, allow to steep for at least 20 minutes.

Drink one cup at a time to help flush excess sodium or relieve fluid retention.

Refrigerate left over tea. It is good warm or cold. It is alkalizing because it is a good source of minerals. Note: Commercial parsley is sprayed to deter pests. Be sure to clean it in a *Thieves Cleaner/Lemon Oil* bath and rinse well.

GREEN "FAST FOOD" SMOOTHIE

(RWR use fruits on plan - sweeten with stevia.)

Nutrient dense leafy greens are rich in alkalizing minerals and live enzymes. Blend raw spinach and romaine lettuce in <u>cold</u> water with fresh ginger, then add 2 scoops of Young Living's *Balance Complete* protein powder. Yum!

Choose kale or collard greens, water to liquify then add fruits like frozen mango and blueberries or pineapple. Romaine lettuce goes well with 1/2 an orange, a bit of fresh ginger (or use ever so little of *Ginger* essential oil) and 1/2 a frozen banana.

SNACKS

Daily snacks are an important part of the RWR plan. Snacks are intended to help your energy and blood sugar level. This is to send the message that you are consistently giving the body what it needs to maintain fuel for your brain and muscles. This will remove stress messages that are created by hunger, and keep your body from feeling the need to go into a protective mode of holding on to fat in case it will be needed for fuel. Do not skip meals, and plan snacks to carry with you if you think your meal will be delayed.

Fruits make ideal snacks for this purpose, because they are digested quickly for muscle and brain energy and they have some fiber that helps to slow their sugar release. Fruits are composed of both sucrose and fructose, which is an easier sugar composition for the body to handle. A person eating according to the CMS plan may choose from a wide variety of colors and textures among the many kinds of fruits available. Variety is key to the CMS plan so it is suggested that many kinds of fruits are eaten instead of staying with just two or three. Eat a few soaked nuts with fruit.

Fruit snacks should be spaced well between meals or at least 20-30 minutes before the next meal. A meal of protein and vegetables will usually take about two hours to clear the stomach. If fruit is eaten before the stomach empties, bloating and gas may result from adding an alkaline fruit to an acid digestive environment in progress. Eating a few soaked nuts with fruit snacks will also slow the digestion of the fruit sugars and provide protein and fats, and can curb true hunger pains.

The RWR fruit list is limited to only four fruits eaten as snacks during the 4 weeks of rapid weight reduction, plus 1 lemon per day if you wish. The fruits are eaten twice a day between meals: 1/2 a medium apple, 1/2 a large grapefruit, 1/2 an orange or 6 strawberries. To follow correct food combining, RWR fruit should always be eaten between meals. Do not peel your apples, but make sure you have washed them well. Grapefruit is known to assist weight loss. Oranges help with stress and are a good source of antioxidants that support immune function. Eat some of the white too, as it is rich in bioflavonoids. Grapefruit and oranges are good as bedtime snacks to help maintain blood sugar.

CMS protein snacks can include 5 or 6 walnuts, 8 soaked almonds, or a tablespoon of pumpkin seeds chewed well till they are liquified before swallowing. RWR protein snacks eaten between meals are 2 ounces of sliced chicken or turkey or one hard boiled egg. A walnut or two or a few soaked almonds won't disrupt your diet chemistry during the four weeks, but if you do not digest nuts well, it's probably best if you wait to eat these.

CMS shakes and smoothies can be made with almond milk, hemp milk, whey protein powder and fresh or frozen (not canned) fruits like peaches, blueberries, blackberries or strawberries. RWR shakes and smoothies being drunk as fruit and whey protein snacks should be prepared with water (or may use a combination of 1/2 water and 1/2 almond or hemp milk - rice milk is too sweet), and an orange or strawberries. Young Living's *Pure Protein Complete, Power Meal* or *Balance Complete* deliver needed protein plus other nutrients and fiber.

On CMS there are ready-made snacks that you may find at your local health food and grocery stores. You must read labels to avoid bad fats and sugars. You don't want your snacks defeating your purpose, and you still need the nutrients that fruit snacks provide. It's best to stick with them, but if you are desperate for more variety, need the packaged convenience, and if you are confident in reading labels then look for snacks that are between 70 and 100 calories and have a good protein profile. Divide a calorie-rich snack bar if it is over 100 calories.

RWR and CI folks beware! Don't think the old favorites of dry popcorn or rice cakes will be your snacks. These foods are high on both Glycemic Index and Glycemic Loading because they are well along the path of conversion from starch to sugar by being "popped." This is true of all popped grains like puffed wheat or crispy rice. If you are looking for something drier and heavier than fruit as a snack, then occasionally, during the four weeks, make the cinnamon toast recipe made with organic coconut oil.

Realize that this will count as one of your two starch servings for the day. However, it really is a welcomed treat with a cup of herb tea. As a side note: use ground cinnamon whenever it seems appropriate, such as on baked acorn squash or sliced apples. It is known to help with regulating blood sugar.

CMS allows small portions of hard cheese, such as a one-inch cube of Monterey Jack or white cheddar which can satisfy as a protein/fat snack with some green grapes or a few apple slices. RWR limits fats and dairy, but one dairy food that may be eaten is plain Greek yogurt. Five to six ounces may be eaten as breakfast or 2 ounces as a snack with a few strawberries. CMS, try it with 1/4 cup of blueberries.

Be creative with 2 ounce portions of protein foods for snacks. Also, stay alert when reading cook books or other literature to find meal and snack recipes.

In his article, "Does Eating More Frequent Meals Really Rev Up Your Metabolism?" Dr. Joseph Mercola, DO, counsels, "Snacks, as long as they're nutritious, of course, could also help you avoid overeating later because you're ravenous and eat too quickly once you do sit down for a meal. It may also help you stick to healthier food choices, since many people tend to reach for fast food or quick and easy processed foods when they are tired and hungry."[32]

YOUNG LIVING ESSENTIAL OILS
SECTION 6: Table 3 - SNACKS

The Ningxia wolfberry has the highest known levels of immune-boosting polysaccharides; four times the beta-cryptoxanthin than the # 2 source, red hot chili peppers; three times the vitamin C of oranges; five times the potassium of bananas; and 91 percent more fiber than raw oats.[33]

This is the only fruit juice for CMS, but dilute 1 ounce with 4 to 6 ounces of water. (RWR avoid until you cycle back to CMS.)

Thieves Lozenges have the sweet flavor of *Peppermint, Lemon* and other natural sugars with *Thieves* essential oil blend. Allow one to dissolve slowly in your mouth for soothing relief when needed for a bit of a pick up.

Support your body's natural defenses with *Super C Chewable* tablets when you want to have a little bite of something to chew as a snack. They are enhanced with minerals, bioflavonoids, and pure *Orange* essential oil.

Healthy snack bars are: *Wolfberry Crisp Bar, YL Manna Apricot Bars* and *YL Manna Apple-Cinnamon.* CMS limit to 1/2 a bar. (RWR limit to 1/4 bar or avoid until you cycle back to CMS.)

CMS
Section 6: Table 4 - PROTEIN & FAT SNACKS

Walnuts, raw (soaked 4 hours): 1/8 cup or 1/2 ounce =
6 to 7 walnut halves

Almonds, raw (soaked 8 to 12 hours): 1/4 cup or 1 ounce =
15 almonds

Cashews, raw (soaked 4 hours): 1/4 cup or 1 ounce =
8 to 9 whole cashews

Brazil nuts (high fat), raw (soaked 8 to 12 hours): 1/8 cup or
1/2 ounce = 3 whole nuts

CHEW NUTS UNTIL LIQUID BEFORE SWALLOWING!

Section 7

"Your chances of success
in any undertaking
can always be measured
by your belief in yourself."

~ Robert Collier

Motivational Speaker

DEFINITIONS OF TERMS

Throughout this book, terms like carbohydrates, protein and fats are central to the theme and to understanding the actual plans. Generally, the standard by which we are to measure or define these "scientific" terms, that belong to the domain of nutrition, is set by our government. Those of us who lean toward the "all natural" approach to diet and nutrition are not always on the same page because we believe there are unseen, energetic forces and universal Laws of Nature at work that must be acknowledged which science cannot quantify.

Personally, when it comes to health, I prefer to seek help from someone who is more specifically a consumer health advocate. Dr. Bernard Jensen, PhD, has been one such advocate and Teacher whose philosophy of natural nutrition for a vital life was an example of this type of wisdom. However, he did not ignore the "science" of nutrition in practicing the "art" of natural nutrition. After all, not all that is deemed "natural" is necessarily fit for human consumption. Just as not all that is considered of value by the scientific community is fit for humans either. Let us be discerning.

Scientists study what they can see and ask, "What is life?" as Dr. Jensen explains, "The life that makes up the unseen part of our environment is more multitudinous and universal and influential on our lives than that which is seen." He adds, "They have explored human tissue down to the single cell and its process, but exactly what makes that cell alive is not known... The power of unfolding any physical thing that we may see is found in the Vital Force that operates in the plant, the animal or the man, and it is that force which vitalizes the seed and causes it to sprout and to grow... It is natural law that keeps us in the shape we are in. By working with this universal force we can make changes through the matter, the food, the sunshine we live in, and the good habits we keep."[33]

As you read the definitions of terms of the macro elements that comprise foods and the CMS/RWR plans, realize that it is the Vital Force of nature's handiwork that we hope to enhance to restore intuition about the energetic force in our foods and our thoughts for greater freedom of health. The definitions of terms presented in this book are projected through the prism of these beliefs:

- ▸ God created the Universe and all that is.

- ▸ The "herbs of the field" were created to be our "meat" and our "medicine."

- ▸ Fruits, vegetables and therapeutic-grade essential oils are "herbs of the field."

- ▸ Each of us must take personal responsibility for our own health care.

- ▸ Mind/body/emotions are intimately connected, especially where food and eating are concerned.

- ▸ With awareness we can learn to choose the best for our families.

- ▸ Our bodies have innate wisdom to heal and correct imbalances.

- ▸ An ounce of prevention is truly worth a pound of cure.

- Foods known to be low glycemic, or have a low glycemic effect on the blood sugar, can help prevent or lessen blood sugar imbalances.

- Moderate amounts of "fit fats" are necessary for health, and do not cause us to be fat.

- We must have a limited amount of salt each day - unrefined, mineral sea salt is preferred.

- Our blood is salty because it must remain at an alkaline pH.

- "The life of the flesh is in the blood."[34]

- Chemical messengers or neurotransmitters from the central command center of the brain (hypothalamus) are responsible for thirst, hunger, appetite control and satiety. These messages are effected by lifestyle choices.

- Plenty of filtered water is needed every day for optimal brain function, joints and skin hydration, blood viscosity, and to maintain a healthy weight.

- Synthetic chemical- and oil-based cosmetics are absorbed into our bodies, and must be metabolized and processed to be eliminated or they are stored in fat.

- We must be educated to avoid certain foods such as high fructose corn syrup (HFCS), "unfit fats," MSG- and GMO-containing foods and beverages.

- Medicinal drugs have been developed through the study and extraction of isolated factors from botanicals and other natural elements, and are usually void of the micro elements of the original botanicals.

▸ Drugs often target symptoms rather than deliver nutritional elements for the body to use to heal itself. (Hopefully, they are only needed on a temporary basis.)

▸ Sweet foods may be defined as expansive and elicit opposite, balancing urges or cravings for salty foods that contract.

▸ Whole foods carry micro and macro elements that our bodies know how to process for our benefit.

▸ Processed foods, though often convenient, lack whole food elements.

▸ The food industry is Big Business, and the outcome of their financial report is what stockholders are generally concerned about; therefore decisions on the food supply are likely more about business than the nation's health.

▸ "Organic" has become a commercial marketing term causing some to doubt the true value of products described as "organic" or "natural."

▸ Organic foods can be healthier if you get real organic foods, grown by real farmers you can trust. (Talk with growers at your local Farmer's Market.)

▸ True organic foods taste better. The foods have complete nutrient profiles, and will be free of toxic agricultural chemicals.

▸ Being grateful, forgiving and positive about life relieves undue stress.

▸ If we surround ourselves with positive, uplifting people, places and beauty, we will become uplifting and a positive influence and blessing to others.

▸ We can train our hearts and eyes to see beauty all around us.

▸ I believe that when the student is ready, the teacher will appear.

PURE WATER

As we all know, water is crucial to survival. In his book, <u>Your Body's Many Cries for Water - You Are Not Sick, You Are Thirsty!</u>, Dr. F. Batmanghelidj, MD, asks and answers the question:

Q. "Why are 30 percent of Americans over weight?"

A. "Because of a most basic confusion! They don't know when they are thirsty; they also don't know the difference between 'fluids' and 'water.'"[35]

He teaches, "The truth is that dehydration can cause disease. Everyone knows that water is 'good' for the body. They seem not to know how essential it is to one's well-being. They do not know what happens to the body if it does not receive its daily need of water."[36]

Water mechanisms that work within body systems, like the endocrine and digestive systems, are very critical to well-being for weight reduction as well as other conditions that may be experienced because of chronic dehydration. Dr. Batmanghelidj explains how the "central control system" in the brain for hunger and thirst are related, and that most overweight people feel the sensation of hunger when their body is signaling that it is thirsty. He counsels patients seeking to reduce weight to be well hydrated before meals so that the hypothalamus satiety control messages are recognized, signaling they are no longer hungry and consequently will stop eating. Also, he counsels that, "Other fluids don't count," and explains that there are detrimental, long-term consequences on the sensitivities of the control system of the brain and liver that become deranged from drinking sodas and fluids containing artificial sweeteners.

One way to break puffiness or fluid-retention is to drink more water. The kidneys are involved in maintaining fluid balance in the body as well as cellular sodium/ potassium balance. Dehydration causes the body to hold on to sodium as a protective mechanism that involves our blood and vital systems. Dehydration is a major stress for the body, and it musters many forces, using a good portion of our energy to ensure that this high priority for the blood system is maintained. Our blood needs water and natural sodium found in foods like celery and high potassium foods like parsley and watermelon.

You may be wondering if flavoring your water with essential oils has any drawbacks. I know of none. Studying the osmotic and energetic action of essential oils will allow you to decide the answer to this question. Water is one source of oxygen for the body, but if chronically dehydrated, the cell membranes of the body may not be as permeable and receptive to hydration. Essential oils help facilitate the process for greater absorption and appear to increase oxygen or at least increase the utilization of the oxygen that is already in the body.

Due to Dr. Batmanghelidj's recommendations, I began drinking at least 1/2 my body weight in ounces of water every day, and have included it here as a major consideration for CMS and RWR. Also, his book is very informative about how it is that drinking pure water is preventive of so many heath concerns. He has an interesting discussion of the physiology of sodium, blood pressure and fluid retention or edema. If I had any of these concerns, I'd want to study his book.

Other concerns include the many chemicals that are found in our water supplies. We can filter our drinking water to help remove the chlorine and fluoride, (thought to be detrimental to thyroid function), but what about our bath and shower water? You may wish to investigate the feasibility of installing filters on the main water entrance line. Also, there are shower head attachments that can be filled with Epsom salts (as a medium for essential oils too) that help to lessen the chemical load, or at least we can add Epsom salts, and gentle essential oils to bath water.

CMS & RWR
Section 7: Table 1 - WATER

...Did you know, bottled water may not be as healthy a source of water for you to drink then if you were to simply filter your own tap water?

...Also, remember that drinking water lubricates your joints & keeps your skin moist.

...Did you also know that plastic bottles are more than an environmental disaster? There is a good chance that chemicals called xenoestrogens have leached into waters bottled in plastics; especially if the bottle has been left in the sun or a hot car. These estrogens mimic our own estrogen, causing disruption of our natural endocrine system processes.

YOUNG LIVING ESSENTIAL OILS
Section 7: Table 2 - FLAVORED WATER

Tip from Peggy Martin
Young Living Independent Distributor

Each day prepare 2 empty *NingXia Red* bottles as follows:
Put *Grapefruit* essential oil drops in one and
Peppermint essential oil drops in the other.
Fill with filtered water, 4 cups each, 64 ounces total
Drink throughout the day.
NOTE: Do not put essential oils in plastic water bottles.

Thanks to Peggy for this healthy recycling use
of the *NingXia Red* one-liter bottles.

SALT - THE FOOD ELEMENT SODIUM

Salt is essential to good health, but not all salts are the same. You must learn to distinguish the difference between the value of unrefined sea salt, Himalayan (from pristine areas of the high Himalayan Mountains), Celtic salt or Real Salt (which is sourced from the Great Salt Lake in Utah) and devitalized table salt. When you read the sodium profile on packaged foods, the manufacturers are referring to sodium of the sodium chloride, table salt variety. Otherwise, if sea salt is used these brands will indicate that it is sea salt because they know that consumers, like us, will appreciate that fact. Celtic sea salt is about 84 percent sodium chloride. Himalayan salt contains eighty-plus minerals and trace elements and is thought to be the purest, nutritionally complex salt.

Have you noticed how your tears, blood, and perspiration are salty? The extra cellular spaces, or area around our cells, are to be bathed in a sodium bath. Potassium is the element within the cells, and when all is in balance we experience the energy potential each little cellular battery produces - the spark of life. Scripture tells us, "The life of the flesh is in the blood."[37] Our blood must also remain at a slightly alkaline pH. This is a very high priority for the body, so learning to distinguish which salt is best for you becomes a wonderful partnership for greater health. We must eat salt from either electron-rich, alkaline, crystalline unrefined sea salt and/or from foods that are known to be a good source of readily available nutritional sodium.

Some fond memories on my wellness journey are of being taught by Dr. Bernard Jensen, PhD, and how he maintained such a gentle manner while imparting important precepts. I had the great fortune to be treated and study with him at his Hidden Valley Ranch in Escondido, California. I can still hear him say, "The stomach is a sodium organ. You will find that whey is one of the best foods for the stomach, most especially goats' milk whey." He spoke of the blood and the need to have food-grade sodium to neutralize the acids so the body did not have to draw mineral ions from its own tissues to maintain blood alkalinity. He explained sodium chloride and how stress is so very detrimental to the digestive process because stress uses up chlorine and, when we eat, the cells of the stomach release hydrogen molecule-for-molecule according to the amount of chlorine molecules that are available at the time of digestion to make hydrochloric acid, which is necessary to break down protein for digestion. He'd tell us that there are so many things of importance to do to help ourselves and others, but this is of great importance. We must cleanse out the taste for devitalized table salt. We must avoid it and flush it from our systems so we can truly appreciate what energetically alive sodium crystals taste and feel like in our bodies. He'd say, "You are the salt of the earth, you were meant to eat the salt of the earth, there is life in it." He would also gently counsel, "You must help people to feel better so then they can BE better."

Sodium is needed by the body for water regulation, nervous system and muscle activity, adrenal gland function, etc. However, both CMS and RWR insist that table salt be banned from your presence. In his book, The No Grain Diet, Dr. Joseph Mercola, DO, explains, "Ordinary table salt contains chemical additives and is processed at over 1200 degrees, which changes its chemical structure, and therefore, it should not be used often."[38] He also counsels, "If you need to avoid salt due to high blood pressure or kidney problems, lemon crystals and lemon pepper are good replacements, giving your food a mouthwatering zing."[39]

It is suggested you measure a little salt to regulate how much you use every day. The suggested daily amount noted by the National Academy of Sciences is 1/2 teaspoon, which is no doubt a measure of common table salt. Use sea salt instead. They report, "On average, Americans consume more than 3,400 milligrams of sodium - the amount in about 1.5 teaspoons of salt - each day. The recommended maximum daily intake of sodium -- the amount above which health problems appear - is 2,300 milligrams per day for adults, about 1 teaspoon of salt. The recommended adequate intake of sodium is 1,500 milligrams per day, and people over 50 need even less."[40]

For CMS and RWR purposes, we measure between 1/4 and 1/2 teaspoon of unrefined sea salt into a little bowl each morning and sprinkle pinches of it from the bowl through the day's meals as a condiment. When a bit is left by the end of the day, and you tolerate sea salt, it can be added to a full glass of water to become a mineral-rich, purifying solution to drink.

SUGARS & SWEETENERS

Human physiology is designed to use sugars to move our muscles and to create brain energy. Our original design has conditioned us to desire foods that taste sweet so we will fulfill this critical energy supply. We were also originally designed to use the complex sugars that are found in botanicals such as fruits, berries, and other vegetation. Complex sugars are usually found structured handily within the fiber of plant tissues. When eaten, these sugars are gradually released from the fiber during digestion, and not as likely to increase the demand on pancreas function like refined sugar is known to do.

In contrast to complex sugars that nature has packaged in fiber, processed, white or brown table sugar are chemically simple sugars. This sugar breaks down quickly during digestion and can give the blood sugar a quick lift. Natural cane or beet sugar is actually preferable, as far as sugar chemistry goes, to the all-pervasive fructose now found in thousands of products with high-fructose corn syrup (HFCS).

The News at Princeton University reported "A sweet problem... Princeton researchers find that high-fructose corn syrup prompts considerably more weight gain. They have found that in diets with equal calories, high-fructose corn syrup leads to significantly more weight gain than regular sugar... It increases risk for high blood pressure, heart disease, cancer, and diabetes appreciably more than sugar."[41]

Table sugar may be a better choice than HFCS, but it is still not the best sweetener for us. So, what is best? That depends on the individual, but during CMS and RWR, sugars of all stripes are avoided. This allows the body to cleanse and remove the stress that simple sugars cause. After RWR, I gradually reintroduced Young Living's organic *Blue Agave,* some maple syrup and a little date sugar in limited amounts.

Honey is nature's original, very concentrated sweetener so a little goes a long way, but still it will be prudent to delay its use until you have given your body the chance to dampen down cravings for sugars. *Blue Agave* from Young Living is a natural sweetener I'd use as an alternative to refined sugar or artificial sweeteners, because its Glycemic Index score is low even though agave is a fructose sugar.

Understanding the health implications of sugars is very important to your weight reduction goals. It is the main issue, and the reason I have stressed that you seriously consider making it a number one priority to cleanse your body from all sugars except for the natural sugars you will receive from vegetables, limited starches and fruits. If you wish to delve deeper into studies about this, read about the study created by Emory University and the American Heart Association. They "found that the more added sugars the (study participants) ate, the lower their good cholesterol, and the higher their triglycerides, blood fats that also increased risk for diabetes and heart disease at elevated levels."[42] The American Heart Association links too much added sugar and heart disease, prompting their recommendations to 'specific limits of 6 teaspoons daily for women and 9 teaspoons daily for men. The American average is more than 22 teaspoons daily.'"[43]

Again, it is important to realize that sugars in fresh fruits and vegetables are not the problem. (Unless you are

Carbohydrate Intolerant.) The Nutrition Facts labels on all packaged foods (the chart listing calories, protein, fats, etc.) will list the sugar content of that food item according to quantity, but know that they don't separate added sugars from naturally occurring ones. If sugar appears near the top of the ingredients list then it is a large percentage of the contents. If the package or bottle label lists any of the following sugars, put it back on the shelf and find or create a healthy alternative: cane sugar, beet sugar, cane juice, corn syrup, maple syrup, molasses, honey, high-fructose corn syrup, or brown rice syrup.

YOUNG LIVING ESSENTIAL OILS
Section 7: Tabel 3 - SUGARS & SWEETENERS

Did you know that cinnamon helps with sugar metabolism? Use ground cinnamon often or try barely a drop of *Cinnamon Bark* essential oil. Make coconut oil-cinnamon toast with stevia herbal extract. The fiber of your whole grain toast will help slow down the digestion of the sugar.

A smoothie treat we like is to put 1/2 teaspoon of ground cinnamon with a cup of organic almond milk, 1 scoop of Young Living whey, *Pure Protein Complete*, and 1 ripe banana. Banana is higher on the Glycemic Index as it delivers three sugars: sucrose, fructose and glucose. So, the fruit sugar of a banana can be a good thing when working or playing hard. You may find that the addition of cinnamon will help balance blood sugar. You might also add one or two tablespoons of raw, organic peanut or almond butter in the smoothie for the extra protein. Avoid banana while on RWR.

Young Living's *Blue Agave* is low on the Glycemic Index. It may be used in baking in the place of honey or sugar. Mix with coconut oil and cinnamon as a spread for pancakes or whole grain toast. *Stevia Extract* is a dietary supplement that supports pancreas function and helps to maintain normal blood sugar levels.* One serving has a Glycemic Index of zero.

These statements have not been evaluated by the Food and Drug Administration.

While seeking balance and to offer suggestions for healthy substitutes to the physical burdens sugar can cause, I've recently heard of yacon syrup, which is claimed to be a sugar substitute that is not detrimental to health, so I thought it would be worth investigating.

Coincidental to my bit of research about yacon syrup, and much to my delight, pictures were shown at the Young Living 2010 Annual Convention of yacon growing on the Young Living Essential Oils farm, Finca Botanica Aromatica, in Guayaquil, Ecuador. (I tasted it at Convention in a delightful Wu Long tea that had been sweetened with yacon from the farm.)

I found it to be smooth with no bitterness, and though it is zero on the Glycemic Index it was almost too sweet for my taste buds - perhaps because I've been avoiding sugars. However, the tea would be a perfect fit for our CMS and RWR programs so naturally I hope to see it added to the Young Living product line. It provides several health benefits and is being considered to be hopeful for diabetes prevention.

Another natural food-source sweetener is date sugar. Just remember that the taste of any concentrated sweet such as date sugar, herbal stevia (sweet leaf), agave syrup or yacon syrup will begin to make the liver ready for the body to use sugar as fuel. But, since we want the liver to rest, we limit sugars of all kinds to our fruits and vegetables and these few healthier sources for our initial cleansing period on CMS, and totally restrict all added sugars for the three weeks of RWR.

It feels so good to be free of sugar and carbohydrate addiction. I promise it is worth the effort to do this for yourself. Don't be in too much of a hurry to go back to the sweets - especially if you find you are Carbohydrate Intolerant. Just remember that excess sugar of any kind gets stored as fat if it is not used by the brain and muscles soon after digestion, and if the body is using ingested sugars as fuel, then it is not drawing on stored fat for energy. You will be able to adequately satisfy your body's need for sugars from the fruit snacks and smoothies you'll be eating as well as from starches and vegetables. Eat your snacks, don't skip meals and get plenty of restful sleep. Of course, if you have any questions about sugars and blood sugar imbalances, it is best to consult with your doctor.

CMS & RWR

SECTION 7: Table 4 - YACON SYRUP

Asking with curiosity I asked, "What is yacon syrup?" months before I knew that Young Living had transplanted some from Peru to the farm in Eucador to research its benefits. My curiosity was answered by eHow Contributing Writer, Christopher Goodwin's description:

"Yacon syrup is a natural sugar substitute grown in the foothills of the Andean Mountain region of South America, and was first used by the ancient Incas...

The enzyme that makes yacon root sweet is FOS, Fructooligosaccharide, 50 percent of yacon plant roots are made up of FOS. The taste of yacon syrup is compared to molasses, caramel and honey. It has a richer stronger taste than regular sugar, and should be used sparingly in recipes...

For weight loss, yacon syrup is extremely low in calories because its main enzyme cannot be retained by the body. Those on diets for cosmetic or health reasons can use yacon syrup without worrying about empty calories...

According to a February 2008 study published in 'Clinical Nutrition Magazine,' it has been shown that yacon syrup is beneficial to the body when used moderately. It contains bacteria, similar to that found in yogurt, and helps to regulate the digestive system... Yacon syrup also does not pose any of the potential health risks that some artificial sweeteners do."[45]

FATS - THE FIT AND THE UNFIT

Like sweeteners, people love fats. Fats lend lots of flavor but, more than that, certain fats are essential to our health. We are designed to prefer fats to ensure that we provide them in our diet as they're critical to the brain and central nervous system.

Friendly, fit fats are found in eggs, avacado, certain cold-water fish, organic butter, organic coconut oil and organic virgin olive oil. You will also get some of the fats you need from nuts such as almonds, Brazil nuts, cashews, pecans, macadamia, and walnuts. Seeds, too, are little powerhouses of energy, but both your nuts and seeds are best if germinated or soaked to release the growth inhibitors and give their enzymes a boost for more complete digestion and utilization of their nutrients. Use soaked golden flax seeds, chia seeds, alfalfa seeds, radish seeds, sunflower seeds, and mung seeds, among others. Change the germination water regularly, and allow some of your seeds to make delicious sprouts that can be tossed on and into everything.

Raw cheeses, raw organic nut butters and Tahini (sesame paste) are more options, but while on RWR, restrict their use until after you've completed the month. Nut butters are almond, cashew and peanut. Peanuts should be carefully investigated because they are prone to a toxic mold that is dangerous to humans and animals. Avoid this aflatoxin by purchasing peanut products that you trust.

Then there are the unfit fats. Sometimes you will hear them called the "bad" fats. Actually, in their raw, pure state these fats could be beneficial, but unfortunately they have become so popular that they are found in thousands of prepared foods, and usually in the form of hydrogenated or trans fatty acids. If we eat out at all, we're sure to be ingesting more than a healthy quota of denatured and sometimes even rancid Omega 6 vegetable seed oils.

Then there are the Omega 6 vegetable oils refined from the seeds of canola, corn, safflower, soy, sunflower, etc. When high heat is used during cooking with these oils, trans fatty acids and free radicals are created. These are the bad "unfit fats" that cause harm to the body. There is the Genetically Modified Organisms issue, too. None of these oils are suggested for either CMS or RWR, but we do need some Omega 6 - so find a brand you trust to use a little now and then in salad dressings or marinades. I use Macadamia Nut oil or a little Safflower oil for this reason. The really bad fats are thought to be the saturated fats found in lard and red meats, but not all sources of saturated fats are harmful - limited ingestion of organic butter, organic coconut oil and avacados are some healthy sources. Just remember what someone probably told you at some time, "Moderation in all things." That is so true when eating fatty foods.

Trans fat is also created when vegetable oils are hydrogenated or partially-hydrogenated by infusing the liquid oils with hydrogen to turn them into a solid form. Food sources include bagels, candies, cakes, pies, cookies, pastries, bisquits, cereals, deep fried foods, fatty meats, soups, margarines, and some salad dressings. You must read labels.

Research reveals that our bodies' engines run best on an equal amount of Omega 3 to Omega 6 fats (EFAs) in a ratio of 1:1, with some Omega 9, too. The inordinate proportions of 6s to 3s is thought to be a sources of inflammation throughout the body. If you've ever experienced a condition with a name that ends in an "itis," then you know first-hand what inflammation feels like. These conditions may indicate an imbalance of too much Omega 6 oils in relation to the amount of Omega 3 Essential Fatty Acids in the diet.

Oil soluable vitamins, A-D-E-K also need quality fats from our diets for proper absorption and utilization. Of special interest to our weight reduction goals is the fact that essential fatty acids are necessary for the production of endrocrine chemical messengers. Many glands are dependent on fat that the body uses to make their appropriate messages to direct their function. The adrenal glands help regulate sugar, minerals and stress, and need fat. Also, too low a fat consumption can cause lowered metabolism. Obviously, even though "fit fat" is good for us, we must be careful to limit the amount we eat as there is more than twice the caloric value in a gram of fat (9) than a gram of carbohydrate (4), except for coconut oil that is digested like carbohydrates and is just over 6 calories per gram.

PROTEIN

Protein means "of first importance." It is needed to rebuild every cell in the body. Quality digested protein plays a major role in nearly every chemical process that affects our physical and mental state. Proteins manufacture enzymes, chemical messengers and antibodies. They are building and repairing foods.

As a general rule, each day we need to eat about 1/2 gram of protein for each pound of ideal body weight. Pregnant women, lactating mothers and teenagers may need from 1/3 to 1/2 more protein than other people of the same weight. If 150 is an ideal weight for someone, this person will need 75 grams per day for optimum health, balanced with a proportionate intake of complex carbohydrates, fiber, water and moderate amounts of fat.

On a long term basis, protein should come from the diet. However, when I need to supplement protein in my diet, I have found it convenient to make protein drinks with any of the three Young Living formulations: *Power Meal, Pure Protein Complete* or *Balance Complete*.

As a side note, no doubt you realize that knowing what to eat and how much to eat for adequate protein is important, but if a person has difficulty digesting protein foods this could require extra care and support to the digestive system. One way to support protein digestion and assimiltion is to supplement your meals with digestive enzymes. There are many enzyme products on the market from which to choose, and our family has tried many brands, but we always come back to Young Living's *Essentialzyme* for the most consistent overall results. Also, if we have eaten something that does not feel just right, we have found that Young Living's *Detoxzyme* clears the discomfort very quickly. We never travel without *Essentialzyme* and *Detoxzyme* in a handy packet.

When one eats protein, the process of breaking it down into amino acids begins in the stomach. There are 20 amino acids, 9 of which are called "essential amino acids" because we must provide them through our diets. The proportion of aminos to each other is another factor in play too, but fortunately we do not have to figure out which foods are delivering what proportion of aminos because our intelligent bodies know when all aminos are present and accounted for, and ready to create new tissues. This fact is another reason eating the variety suggested by CMS works in our favor.

If necessary, the body can use protein to create energy if insufficient levels of fats or carbohydrates have been eaten. However, when carbohydrates like fresh vegetables and whole grains are eaten at a meal with protein, they supply energy to the body, sparing the protein and allowing it to tend to its work of rebuilding tissues. Poor quality proteins will limit the body's ability to create quality tissue. This is where the well-known saying, "You are what you eat," takes shape - literally shapes your body! High quality, well balanced protein provided from a wide variety of the CMS and RWR food categories will create high quality, healthy blood and tissue.

Complete protein foods contain all the amino acids in proper amounts for human use. Meats, fish, poultry, cheese, eggs, yogurt and milk are complete protein foods. The finest protein, and the one which is assigned the hightest biological activity, is the egg. Legumes, grains, vegetables, fruits, nuts and seeds all contain incomplete protein, as they are poorly balanced in amino acid content. What this means is that these foods, if eaten alone, will not supply enough top-grade protein for the tissues. However, when these foods are eaten in combinations, the amino acid balance is improved and the protein quality is increased. These combinations do not have to be at the same meal for the body to ultimately utilize the protein.

Vegetarians who eat nothing of animal origin will find that all whole fruits and vegetables contain protein, and the old theory that some foods must be combined at the same meal to get enough high quality protein in their diets is passe'. However, variety is key. Vegetarians or Vegans will want to choose from all the food categories for a good mix, and not depend on a mono-diet of a few fruits or one or two favorite vegetables, beans or rice.

Then there are the soy-based protein products. Sad to say this is another food source on the avoid list even though it delivers complete protein. Did you know that besides for the documented fact that soy is one of the crops being farmed with Genetically Modified Organisms (corn as well), that it is processed through a bath of hexane which is known to be a neurotoxin?[44] Even if these manufacturing practices were not the norm, soy foods have estrogenic properties that can add to the problem of estrogen dominance and is suspected of contributing to a range of endocrine imbalances.

I mentioned corn in the context of being one of the crops that is most often from Genetically Engineered seed stock. The ramifications of these food industry practices are beginning to reveal some dire consequences to those who have a mind to investigate them. The web site, www.nonGMOshoppingguide.com, is dedicated to collecting data about GMO-free sources that you may print and carry with you to the store. (See Section 10.) About corn though, it is a starch and quickly converts to sugar when digested. On CMS, corn products should be limited to some fresh corn now and then, and RWR should totally avoid all corn for the month.

Wild caught fish is usually a good source of protein, but here again, there are all sorts of warnings about the possibility of contamination by heavy metals and toxic chemicals. Shell fish are good sources too, but remember that they are generally scavengers, and they don't eat very high on the food scale. I'm not fond of shell fish for this reason. Here again, you must decide what is best for you.

In summary, protein foods are of first importance, and they are the foods that we must make the effort to find clean sources. We are very fortunate to be able to find the information we need to decide what to eat and what is best for us and our families. If possible, eat grass fed meats from cattle that live on an open range and eggs gathered from cage-free hens.

Once I heard an individual say that if cattle and other large animals eat nothing but "green" vegetation and grow so very large, then this was reason enough for her to not eat greens! Of course I laughed, but as I thought on this, I realized again how valuable these green herbs of the field are to be able to nourish not only such large bodies of bone, muscle and nerve, but to impart these nutrients to us through the transformations that take place through the wonderful designs of the way digestive and glandular systems have been created. If we ingest our greens before they become a piece of meat or after, earth's most abundant color of chlorophyll-filled, green vegetation is providing for our bones, muscles and nerves. Think about it, whether meat is red or white the best cuts were created from green vegetation.

CMS

Section 7: Table 5 - PROTEIN

...Corn chips and corn tortillas are such favorites for most of us, and they are to be avoided on RWR.

...However, once you are back into a balanced diet on CMS again, find a good brand of corn tortillas and cut them into strips or wedges, spray lightly with some olive oil and lightly sprinkle with sea salt.

...Bake till crisp.

...They brown quickly.

RWR

Section 7: Table 6 - PROTEIN

...Eggs can be used in a variety of ways in meatless dishes for quality protein.

...Add fresh herbs to omelets, frittatas or scrambled eggs.

...Hard boiled, soft boiled, basted (in water) or poached eggs set a good protein profile to add green and red peppers, spinach, mushrooms, tomatoes, sprouts, etc.

CARBOHYDRATES - THE SUGARS & STARCHES

Carbohydrates supply heat and energy from foods that are made up of sugar, starch and fats. The CMS and RWR plans are very high in the consumption of complex carbohydrate plant foods (those in a natural state, totally unrefined). There are two different types of carbohydrates: complex carbohydrates considered to be whole foods and the refined carbohydrates of simple sugars. Starch-based grains, squashes, etc., are also complex carbohydrates. That is, until they undergo processing that renders them into quickly digested simple sugars.

Simple sugars are created when the outer layers of plants are mechanically stripped and refined. The plant's vitamins, minerals, protein and fiber are lost in the process. The foods that results are white sugar, white flour, corn syrup, etc. Foods such as cereals, bakery goods, white rice, instant potatoes, oatmeal, pizzas, and white bread should be avoided. Foods that are prepared with these ingredients are known to give quick energy when needed. However, the long term consequences of relying on simple sugars for energy is detrimental to our health. Blood sugar imbalances are only part of the difficulty from eating simple sugars. For CMS purposes we want to remember that when we eat more energy foods (calories) than what we need at the time, the excess gets stored as fat.

Complex carbohydrates, such as unprocessed fruits, vegetables and whole grains will deliver a longer, slower energy burn along with their nutrients. These are the colorful foods and grains such as quinoa and long grain brown rice that are the basis for meals and snacks when living the CMS lifestyle. Did you know that cooked white rice is higher on the Glycemic Index than a similar sized bowl of ice cream? Yikes! Long grain brown rice is best for CMS and RWR because of its B vitamins and fiber content.

When you begin to avoid the simple sugars of refined carbohydrates, it takes several days, perhaps a week, before you clear these sugars from your body in the first round of cleansing. Once you move past the challenge of any craving urges that might arise, you will begin to see positive results and be encouraged to move toward your goals.

What more need I say about Carbohydrate Intolerance? Even if you do not think this is a concern for you, it would be well to do a simple Google search to read what some "experts" have to contribute to your understanding. If there is a chance that any family member does not digest any of the many forms of sugars found in fresh, whole fruits, vegetables and grains then it will be worth your time and effort. We have found Young Living's *Essentialzyme* to be very beneficial as food enzymes, and their *Carbozyme* is especially formulated to assist with the digestion of starches.

BEVERAGES & HERBAL TEAS

Would you believe you can make a delicious CMS chai latte' at home? It is possible to make a mix of all the spices for homemade chai, but the combination of herbs and spices in Organic India's Marsala Chai is very nice. It is soothing to the palate and the digestion, and it doesn't put a strain on the pocket book or the pancreas with a sugar jolt like the popular versions found at coffee shops. Tulsi Tea (Holy Basil) is another healthful drink from Organic India.

Other teas you might enjoy are organic green teas, Yerba Mate, Chamomile (a relaxing, stress-reducing tea), or an after-dinner Peppermint tea to assist digestion. Being a fan of herb teas, when I heard about the Wu Long Chinese Slimming Tea and what a power-packed antioxidant profile it has, I thought it would be a good one to drink during the RWR segments. It is so valuable to the program, I would drink at least a cup of it each day. A web search will reveal where it is sold.

Fruit juices are restricted on CMS and especially on RWR because they are too high in sugars and usually lack the pulp that would normally allow for a slower release of sugars, as when eating the whole fruit. Vegetable juice like tomato add variety when eating on CMS, and tastes good spiked with lemon juice or apple cider vinegar, but not the best choice for RWR because of high sodium and acidity. However, if you have a juicer and you'd like to make a blood purifying, alkalizing, and building juice full of chlorophyll, try about 4 ounces of my friend, Lori's, Green Drink. (See inset box on page 179.)

Did you know that chlorophyll is only one molecule different from human blood? Chlorophyll's nucleus has magnesium and in our blood is iron. Chlorophyll is an important feature of the CMS/RWR plans for purifying and building our blood, and any program consistently followed requires about three months to cause change in the blood.

Seed or Nut Milks - Make your own protein-rich smoothie milks with sesame seeds, sunflower seeds, or almonds. Soak quality organic seeds or nuts in the refrigerator overnight in filtered water. Drain off the soak water and rinse the nuts or seeds before blending. (I water my house plants with the soak water.) See step-by-step instructions for a variety of nut milks by chef Mandilyn Canistelle in her book, The Raw Food Feast - 7 Days Through the Rainbow.[45] Here's another colorful food theme!

Almond Milk - Use 1 cup soaked almonds to make 1 quart of almond milk. Blend almonds with cold, filtered water long enough to emulsify and liquify the almonds. You may strain the fiber as Mandilyn instructs in her book (then uses it in other creative ways) or leave it in to benefit from the roughage and minerals found in the brown, outer skin. Almond milk is an alkaline beverage, high in protein, easy to absorb and assimilate. It blends well with soups and grain dishes, and it makes an excellent base for fruit smoothies with *Blue Agave* or just a little *Stevia Extract*.

Sunflower or Sesame Seed Milk - Soak 1/4 cup of sesame seeds or sunflower seeds overnight in filtered water. Drain, then place in blender with 2 cups of filtered water. Blend until liquified then strain with a fine wire strainer or a few layers of cheesecloth to remove the hulls. Use as a basis for fruit smoothies with Young Living's *Balance Complete* to help lubricate the intestinal tract for efficient elimination. Sesame seed milk is high in minerals and protein. Sunflower seed milk, made the same way, is high in protein and may be used in any recipe that calls for milk or in smoothies with whey protein like *Pure Protein Complete.* Try either of these milks when adjusting your favorite pancake or waffle recipes for CMS. (See Sesame Waffles recipe in Section 6.)

YOUNG LIVING ESSENTIAL OILS
Section 7: Table 7 - ANTIOXIDANT DRINK

NINGXIA RED NUTRIENT INFUSION

to energize, fortify & replenish the body
NingXia Wolfberries, superfruit plus 5 fruits high in antioxidants
blueberry, pomegranate, apricot, raspberry, grape
and YLTG™ essential oils of *Lemon* and *Orange*

Packaged in 1 liter, glass bottles for optimum nutritional benefit
and 1 oz. travel/sample packets.

Walt's *NingXia Red* Testimonies

I really feel the energy lift within a few minutes after drinking *NingXia Red.* It makes a great smoothie in water with *Balance Complete* and an orange. Also, I am able to drive many more hours on a road trip as long as I drink *NingXia Red* along the route. Thank you Young Living for *NingXia Red*! I drink it every day.

I began wearing prescription sunglasses especially for driving sometime in my 40s. I noticed in my late 60's that my glasses were giving me a headache each time I'd wear them. I had been drinking *NingXia Red* for several months, and had heard that it was good for eye health. At the time, I didn't connect the two until I visited my eye doctor and learned that my eyes had returned to even better than 20/20. Now I'm in my 70's and I've not needed prescription sunglasses since.
-- Walt Anderson, Arvada, CO

CMS & RWR
Section 7: Table 8 - PURE WATER

THE BEST BEVERAGE FOR THE BEST HYDRATION

...Drink 1-2 glasses of pure, *room temperature* water <u>first thing</u> each day to hydrate before drinking anything else...especially before drinking fruit juice or drinking dehydrating beverages like coffee or black tea. This is the BEST way to hydrate while there is nothing else competing with the water.

...Drink at least a full cup of water 10-15 minutes before meals to give a sense of fullness as well as help when your body gives clear cues that you are full so you stop eating sooner.

...Drink just enough water at meals to facilitate digestion of heavier foods and to take your mealtime supplements.

...Drinking cool-to-cold water between meals burns calories as the body heats it to around 98.6 degrees.

...Drinking iced water during meals can interfere with and slows digestion.

...Drink water during exercise.

...Make it a habit to carry your own filtered water in environmentally safe containers.

RWR
Section 7: Table 9 - BEVERAGES

Lori's Green Drink

...Wash and cut ingredients then juice them together: 1 apple, 1/2 lemon with peel, 1 small knob of ginger root, 3 to 4 kale leaves, 3 to 4 Swiss chard leaves, 2 stalks of celery, parsley & enough Romaine lettuce leaves to make 4 to 5 ounces.

...Thanks to Lori McMaster for her version of this cleansing & fortifying green drink.

Chai Latte'

...Pour boiling water over favorite brand Chai like Organic India Marsala Chai & steep until rich, but still hot.
...Sweeten with liquid Stevia to taste.
...Add nut milk such as almond or seed milk of choice.
...Whip together to froth or use special appliance that heats & froths hot drinks.

Walt's Smoothie

...In smoothie maker or blender put 1 cup of water, chipped ice, a peeled & seeded orange, *Balance Complete* and 1 to 2 ounces of *NingXia Red*. Add 1 drop of *Orange* essential oil if you wish.

Blend & enjoy!

Drink Your Salad Greens

The Green "Fast Food" Smoothie on page 141 is a quick way to drink fresh greens. *Balance Complete* protein powder and a drop of stevia (if needed) make a surprisingly tasty between meals snack.

Section 8

"Our bodies are made up of trillions
of living cells, and the cell is
the basic composite of life.
All life takes place at the cellular level.
The cells group together to form tissues.
Tissues group together to form organs.
The organs group together to form
systems.
The systems group together to form the
body."

~ Ronald Glasses, MD

BODY SYSTEMS

Our body systems are so intimately related that whatever affects one will affect all other systems. It is my hope that the following Body Systems[46] lists will help you realize the responsibility we have to feed, nurture, and carefully care for the wonderfully made body in which we live and move and have our Being. The body systems are integral to not only the physical body, but find expression in the psychological and energetic bodies that we must also nourish.

*CIRCULATORY SYSTEM

STRUCTURE: Heart, blood vessels, blood.

FUNCTION: Distribution of oxygen and nutrients to cells, transportation of carbon dioxide and wastes from cells, acid-base balance, regulation of body temperature, formation of blood clots.

FOODS: garlic, wheat germ, chlorophyll, alfalfa sprouts, buckwheat, sun-dried olives, watercress.

HERBS: hawthorne berries, cayenne, ginger, garlic, poke root, sassafras, burdock, echinacea, red clover, oat straw.

ESSENTIAL OILS: *Cinnamon Bark, Clary Sage, Cypress, Goldenrod, Helichrysum, Orange, Palo Santo, Rosemary, Ylang Ylang.*

*DIGESTIVE SYSTEM

STRUCTURE: Gastrointestinal tract with exception of large colon (eliminative). Salivary glands, liver, gall bladder, and pancreas.

FUNCTION: Mechanical and chemical (enzymatic) breakdown of foods for cellular use.

FOODS: papaya, chlorophyll, spinach, sun-dried olives, chard, celery, kale, beet greens, whey, shredded beet, watercress, yogurt and kefir.

HERBS: alfalfa, aloe vera, anise, burdock, comfrey, cayenne, ginger, fennel, papaya, peppermint, slippery elm.

ESSENTIAL OILS: *Basil, Coriander, Dill, Fennel, Ginger, Grapefruit, Ledum, Lemon, Lemongrass, Myrrh, Ocotea, Orange, Patchouli, Peppermint, Spearmint, Tangerine, Tarragon.*

*ELIMINATIVE SYSTEM

STRUCTURE: Kidneys and large colon.

FUNCTION: Completion of nutrient absorption, manufacture of certain vitamins, formation and elimination of feces and urine.

FOODS: all squash, chia seed, flaxseed, green and yellow vegetables, yogurt & kefir, acidophilus, bran, grapes, whey, parsley, psyllium seed, berries, sprouts, yellow cornmeal.

HERBS: psyllium seed, aloe vera, cayenne, black walnut, flaxseed, garlic, slippery elm, Cascara sagrada, senna, barberry, golden seal.

ESSENTIAL OILS: *Basil, Fennel, Fir, Ginger, Lavender, Lemon, Lemongrass, Melaleuca, Mt. Savory, Myrrh, Myrtle, Nutmeg, Oregano, Orange, Spearmint, Tangerine, Tarragon.*

*GLANDULAR SYSTEM

STRUCTURE: Hypothalamus, pineal, pituitary, thyroid and parathyroids, thymus, adrenals, pancreas, ovaries, testes.

FUNCTION: Regulation of body activities through the transportation of chemical messengers by the circulatory system.

FOODS: Sea vegetables, kelp, dulse, swiss chard, turnip greens, egg yolks, wheat germ, lecithin, sesame seed butter, seeds and nuts, raw goat milk.

HERBS: Kelp, dulse, cinnamon, ginseng, dong quai, licorice, echinacea, golden seal, dandelion.

ESSENTIAL OILS: *Chamomile (Roman), Clary Sage, Dill, Fennel, Frankincense, Geranium, Jasmine, Myrrh, Myrtle, Ocotea, Patchouly, Sage, Spearmint, Spruce.*

*RESPIRATORY SYSTEM

STRUCTURE: Lungs, bronchial and sinuses.

FUNCTION: Regulation of oxygen uptake and carbon dioxide removal through respiration and the circulatory system.

FOODS: avocados, blackberries, Brussels sprouts, cabbage, celery, clam broth, cucumber, dates, eggs, endive, fish roe, goat whey, garlic, mangoes, oatmeal, onions, pineapple, salad greens, spinach, tomatoes.

HERBS: alfalfa, boneset juniper berries, lemongrass, licorice, oat straw, parsley, raspberry, wheat straw.

ESSENTIAL OILS: *Clove, Eucalyptus, Eucalyptus Blue, Hyssop (w/carrier oil), Idaho Balsam Fir, Galbanum, Geranium, Marjoram, Melaleuca, Myrtle, Peppermint, Pine, Ravensara, Spearmint, Spikenard, Spruce, White Fir.*

*INTEGUMENTARY

STRUCTURE: Skin, hair, nails, oil and sweat glands.

FUNCTION: Regulation of body elimination of waste, temperature, pressure and pain reception.

FOODS: Goat milk, black bass, rye, sea vegetables, avocados, grapes, whey, apples, cucumbers, millet, rice bran, sprouts.

HERBS: Oat straw, shavegrass, horsetail, aloe vera, burdock.

ESSENTIAL OILS: *Cedarwood, Elemi, Frankincense, Geranium, Lavender, Lemon, Lemongrass, Melaleuca, Rose, Rosemary, Rosewood, Sandalwood.*

*LYMPHATIC SYSTEM

STRUCTURE: Spleen, thymus, appendix, tonsils, lymph nodes, lymph vessels and fluid.

FUNCTION: Filtration of blood, production of white blood cells, immune defenses, return of protein to cardiovascular system.

FOODS: apples, leafy vegetables, watercress, celery, okra.

HERBS: burdock, echinacea, blue flag, poke root, golden seal, cayenne, mullein, black walnut.

ESSENTIAL OILS: *Cinnamon Bark, Cistus, Clove, Frankincense, Hyssop, Juniper, Lemon, Lemongrass, Melaleuca, Melissa, Mt. Savory, Myrtle, Oregano, Rosemary, Sandalwood, Tangerine, Thyme, Wild Tansy.*

*MUSCULAR SYSTEM

STRUCTURE: All muscular tissue in the body.

FUNCTION: Facilitation of body movement, production of heat, maintenance of body posture.

FOODS: Meat proteins, olives, rye, lima beans, rice bran, bananas, sprouts, watercress, complementary proteins (grains, legumes, etc.), apples.

HERBS: Juniper berries, rosemary, tansy, horseradish, wild cabbage, kelp, dulse, watercress, horsetail, black walnut.

ESSENTIAL OILS: *Basil, Chamomile (Roman), Copaiba, Elemi, Eucalyptus, Helichrysum, Idaho Balsam Fir, Juniper, Lavender, Lemon, Lemongrass, Marjoram, Oregano, Palo Santo, Peppermint, Spruce, White Fir, Wintergreen.*

*NERVOUS SYSTEM

STRUCTURE: Brain, spinal cord, nerves and sensory organs such as the eye and ear.

FUNCTION: Regulation of body function through nerve impulses. Sensory perception and motor response.

FOODS: Egg yolks, meat and complimentary proteins, kale, celery, fish, raw goat milk, nutritional yeasts, tryptophan.

HERBS: Valerian, hops, scullcap, lobelia, lady's slipper.

ESSENTIAL OILS: *Cedarwood, Chamomile (Roman), Geranium, Jasmine, Lavender, Melissa, Nutmeg, Sandalwood, Spruce, Valerian, Vetiver, Ylang Ylang.*

*REPRODUCTIVE SYSTEM

STRUCTURE: Testes, ovaries, sperm, ova, mammaries.

FUNCTION: Reproduction of the organism.

FOODS: Sesame & pumpkin seeds, seed & nut butters, egg yolk, lecithin, meat & complimentary proteins, goat milk.

HERBS: Black cohosh, licorice, dong quai, ginseng, blessed thistle, blue cohosh, uva ursi, raspberry, squaw vine, chickweed, saw palmetto, false unicorn.

ESSENTIAL OILS: *Chamomile (Roman), Clary Sage, Fennel, Geranium, Jasmine, Myrrh, Myrtle, Ocotea, Patchouly, Ruta, Sage, Spearmint, Spruce.*

*(These statements have not been evaluated by the Food and Drug Administration. These products are not intended to diagnose, treat, cure or prevent any disease.)

THE BODY SYSTEMS MINI SURVEY

Name_____Age_____Date_____

Score each statement with the number that PRESENTLY
applies the most.

ALMOST NEVER = 1   OCCASIONALLY = 2
OFTEN = 3   MOST OF THE TIME = 4

#1 CIRCULATORY*
1A. Cold hands and/or feet ___
1B. Brain fog +___
1C. Fried or high-fat foods 3 X a week or more +___=___

#2 DIGESTIVE*
2A. Heart burn, excessive burning or want
 ice water at meals ___
2B. Intestinal and/or stomach gas
 (burp, etc.) +___
2C. Pains/upset in abdomen or heavy feeling
 in stomach after meals +___=___

#3 ELIMINATIVE*
3A. Less than 2 bowel movements each day,
 and/or low fiber diet ___
3B. Intestinal gas, flatulence, and/or bloating +___
3C. Constipation, and/or hard stools or
 very loose stools +___=___

#4 GLANDULAR*

4A. Sugars, foods containing sugars, sodas, etc.

    3 X a week or more   ____

4B. Caffeine: coffee, black tea, colas, sodas

    3 X a week or more   +____

4C. Low body temperature upon arising in a.m.

    (below 97.6)   +____ = ____

#5 INTEGUMENTARY (hair, skin, nails)*

5A. Dry, brittle nails and/or dry or thinning hair   ____

5B. Acne, rough and/or problem skin   +____

5C. Dry skin that flakes and/or cracks   +____ = ____

#6 LYMPH/IMMUNE*

6A. Lack of energy or fatigued   ____

6B. Catch illnesses easily   +____

6C. Exercise less than 2 X per week or have

    slow or fast metabolism   +____ = ____

#7 MUSCULAR*

7A. Have ever been exposed to pesticides, chemicals

    or mercury amalgams in teeth   ____

7B. Muscle cramps, pains or "Charlie Horse"

    sensations   +____

7C. Muscle weakness, flaccid, "wasting," or

    hard and tense areas   +____ = ____

8 NERVOUS*

8A. Insomnia or restless sleep patterns   ____

8B. Shaky feelings in limbs or elsewhere, sadness,

    feel like crying   +____

8C. Stress and/or pressures in life   +___ =___

9 REPRODUCTIVE*

9A. Difficult monthly cycles or menstrual
   irregularities (females only)   ___
9B. Stress or lack of energy affecting male organs
   (males only)   +___
9C. Lack of interest in sexual activity   +___
9D. Power surges, sweats or intermittent
   low-grade temperature   +___ =___

#10 RESPIRATORY*

10A. Congestion in sinuses and/or lungs   ___
10B. Cough, sinus problems or breathing condition+___
10C. Breathe polluted air and/or smoke
   cigarettes, cigars, pipe, etc.   +___ =___

#11 SKELETAL*

11A. Spine can't hold adjustments   ___
11B. Pain in bones or joints anywhere in the body +___
11C. Growth problems, mineral depletion   +___ =___

#12 URINARY*

12A. History of kidney or bladder problems   ___
12B. Strong odor, or unusual color when urinating +___
12C. Fluid retention or scanty urine   +___ =___

Since you know your own body and your history, if you feel any body systems need extra support, add your own questions and score them accordingly.

NOTE: IF OVER AGE 40, add 1 point to LYMPH/ IMMUNE SYSTEM, + 1 point to CIRCULATORY SYSTEM, and + 1 point to DIGESTIVE SYSTEM

Write scores for each body system in the boxes below then transfer to the table on the next page.

Circle the High Priority Body Systems that scored 9 or above

BODY SYSTEM SCORES
Section 8: Table 1

date	#1	#2	#3	#4	#5	#6	#7	#8	#9	#10	#11	#12

Date each horizontal section. Track 3 months of surveys.

HIGH PRIORITY AREAS are scores of 9 +

MEDIUM PRIORITY AREAS are scores of 4-8

LOW PRIORITY AREAS are scores of 0-3

Transfer High, Medium and Low Priority scores to the Body Systems Worksheet on the next page.

The Body Systems Mini Survey is for your personal assessment information. It is not to be considered comprehensive, prescriptive, or for diagnosis of illness or disease.

BODY SYSTEMS WORKSHEET
Section 8: Table 2

CIRCULATORY, DIGESTIVE, ELIMINATIVE,
GLANDULAR, INTEGUMENTARY, LYMPHATIC,
MUSCULAR, NERVOUS, REPRODUCTIVE,
RESPIRATORY, SKELETAL, & URINARY SYSTEMS

Label the 3 boxes with scores according to priority
from high to low.

High Priority 9 +	Medium Priority 4-8	Low Priority 0-3

See Body Systems lists on page 194
for possible nutritional support.

BODY SYSTEMS SURVEY RESULTS SHEET
and Key to Young Living Products

Name_____Date_____

List ALL HIGH PRIORITY SYSTEMS - score of 9 or above

_____

List ALL MEDIUM PRIORITY SYSTEMS - score of 4 to 8

_____

List ALL LOW PRIORITY SYSTEMS - score of 0 to 3

_____

Review the pages that follow to become educated about the Essential Oils and/or Supplements* thought to be support for each body system and list them on a separate paper. When you list the oils known for enhancing the 3 high priority areas, you may find some repeated in each box. This way you can see that a few oils can benefit several body systems, or you may find a blend with most of the oils that you want to use.

The following product names are examples of Young Living supplements and essential oils that have traditionally been thought to be of nutritional support for the associated body systems. This list is not for diagnoses, prescription or treatment. This is preventive in nature, and not to replace the services of a licensed health care professional.

You must decide what your body will prefer. Find products that fit most of your High Priority systems first, then look to see which ones also appear for support in the Medium and Low lists. These are nutritional so some supplements support multiple systems at once.

BODY SYSTEMS NUTRITIONAL SUPPORT

*CIRCULATORY: *Master Hers/His, Super B, HRT Tincture, CardiaCare, Thyromin, Pure Protein Complete, NingXia Red, Omega Blue, Rehemogen Tincture, & MultiGreens.* EOs: *AromaLife, Awaken, Citrus Fresh, En-R-Gee, Forgiveness, Goldenrod, Harmony, Joy, Motivation, Present Time, Purification, Release, Valor, Cinnamon Bark, Clary Sage, Cypress, Helichrysum, Orange, Palo Santo, Rosemary, Ylang Ylang, Cel-lite Magic Massage Oil & Diffuser.*

*DIGESTIVE: *Alkalime, Cleansing Trio, Balance Complete, Carbozyme, ComforTone, Essentialzyme, Detoxzyme, Digest & Cleanse, ICP, Life 5, NingXia Red, Rehemogen Tincture & MultiGreens.* EOs: *Abundance, Acceptance, Citrus Fresh, Di-Gize, Forgiveness, Harmony, Joy, Peace & Calming, Present Time, Meditation, Release, Valor, Basil, Dill, Fennel, Galbanum, Ginger, Grapefruit, Lemon, Lemongrass, Myrrh, Orange, Ocotea, Peppermint, Spearmint, Spikenard, Tangerine, Tarragon & Diffuser.*

*LYMPH/IMMUNE: *InnerDefense, Cleansing Trio (ComforTone, ICP, Essentialzyme), Life 5, Balance Complete, Super C, Thyromin, ImmuPro, Allerzyme, NingXia Red & MultiGreens.* EOs: *ImmuPower, Joy, Purification, Thieves, Longevity, Valor, Clove, Exodus II, Cinnamon Bark, Cistus, Frankincense, Hyssop, Juniper, Lemon, Lemongrass, Melaleuca, Myrtle, Oregano, Rosemary, Sandalwood, Spruce, Tangerine, Thyme, Wild Tansy & Diffuser. All Young Living oral, skin and hair products to lessen toxic load from using synthetics.*

*URINARY: *Life 5, Cleansing Trio, Master Formula, Essentialzyme, MultiGreens, K&B Tincture. EOs: Abundance, Acceptance, Di-Gize, Hope, Forgiveness, Harmony, Inspiration, Juniper, Peace & Calming, Purification, Myrtle, Fir, Tangerine, Oregano & Mt. Savory.*

*RESPIRATORY: *Cleansing Trio, Life 5, Super B, Super C, SuperCal & MultiGreens. EOs: Acceptance, Valor, Forgiveness, Harmony, M-Grain, PanAway, Breathe Again, Deep Relief, Peace & Calming, Present Time, Purification, Raven, R-C, Release, Sacred Frankincense, Clove, Eucalyptus, Idaho Balsam Fir, White Fir, Galbanum, Hyssop (only w/carrier oil), Myrtle, Marjoram, Melaleuca, Pine, Peppermint, Ravensara, Spruce & Diffuser.*

*ELIMINATIVE/INTESTINAL: *Life 5, Cleansing Trio (ComforTone, ICP, Essentialzyme), Detoxzyme, JuvaTone, ParaFree, Rehemogen Tincture & Super C. EOs: Di-Gize, Forgiveness, Joy, JuvaFlex, JuvaCleanse, GLF, Peace & Calming, Release, Valor, Basil, Fennel, Ginger, Ledum, Myrrh, Nutmeg, Orange, Spearmint, Tangerine, Tarragon & Diffuser.*

*NERVOUS: *MultiGreens, Super B, Master Formula Hers/His, Super C, SuperCal, MegaCal, Sleep Essence, Mineral Essence, Balance Complete, Pure Protein Complete, Power Meal. EOs: Abundance, Acceptance, Clarity, Common Sense, En-R-Gee, Forgiveness, Gentle Baby, Hope, Harmony, Idaho Balsam Fir, Joy, Motivation, M-Grain, PanAway, Deep Relief Roll-On, Peace & Calming, Present Time, Meditation, RutaVaLa, RutaVaLa Roll-On, Valor, White Angelica, Cedarwood, Roman Chamomile, Geranium, Jasmine, Lavender, Nutmeg, Spruce, Valerian & Ylang*

Ylang. Regenolone Cream, Evening Peace Bath & Shower Gel, Relaxation Massage Oil & Diffuser.

*GLANDULAR/REPRODUCTIVE: *Mineral Essence, Master Hers/His, Endogize, Women's Cortistop, ProGen (males), Progessence Plus Serum (females), PD 80/20, MultiGreens, Blue Agave, Stevia Extract, Thyromin, Balance Complete, Prenolone Plus Body Cream, Protec, Progessence Body Cream, Pure Protein Complete, Carbozyme, Estro Tincture, ThermaBurn, Ultra Young Plus Oral Spray & FemiGen. EOs: Abundance, Acceptance, Awaken, Peace & Calming, Dill, Dream Catcher, Forgiveness, Harmony, Hope, Joy, Mister, Motivation, Release, SclarEssence, Sacred Mountain, 3 Wise Men, Valor, White Angelica, Cinnamon Bark, Geranium, Lady Sclareol, Jasmine, Myrrh, Myrtle, Patchouly, Spearmint, Spruce, EndoFlex, Fennel, DragonTime, En-R-Gee, Rose, RutaVaLa, RutaVaLa Roll-On, Thieves, Purification, Clary Sage, Sage & Diffuser.*

*MUSCULAR/SKELETAL: *Master Formula Hers/His, Balance Complete, Pure Protein Complete, Essentialzyme, Polyzyme, MultiGreens, BLM, BeFit, Omega Blue, Power Meal, MegaCal, Mineral Essence, NingXia Red, Sulfurzyme, SuperCal. EOs: AromaSieze, Deep Relief Roll-On, Basil, Elemi, Envision, Grounding, Helichrysum, Hope, Idaho Balsam Fir, Lavender, Marjoram, PaloSanto, Ortho Ease Massage Oil, Ortho Sport Massage Oil, PanAway, Relieve It, Black Pepper, Purification, & Sacred Mountain.*

*INTEGUMENTARY (hair, skin, nails): *Animal Scents Ointment, AromaGuard deodorants, ART Day Activator, ART*

Gentle Foaming Cleanser, ART Night Reconstructor, ART Purifying Toner, Boswellia Wrinkle Cream, Cel-Lite Magic Massage Oil, ClaraDerm, Essential Beauty Serums, Genesis Hand & Body Lotion, Grapefruit Lip Balm, KidScents Bath Gel, KidScents Lotion, KidScents Shampoo, KidScents Tender Tush, LavaDerm Cooling Mist, Lavender Bath & Shower Gel, Lavender Foaming Hand Soap, Lavender Hand & Body Lotion, Lavender Volume Conditioner, Lavender Volume Shampoo, Lavender Lip Balm, Lavender-Rosewood Moisturizing Soap, LemonSage Clarifying Conditioner, LemonSage Clarifiying Shampoo, Lemon-Sandalwood Cleansing Soap, Master Formula Hers/His, Melaleuca-Geranium Moisturizing Soap, Morning Start Bath & Shower Gel, Morning Start Moisturizing Bar Soap, NingXia Red, Omega Blue, Orange Blossom Facial Wash, Peppermint-Cedarwood Bar Soap, Regenolone Moisturizing Cream, Rose Ointment, Rosewood Moisturizing Conditioner, Rosewood Moisturizing Shampoo, Sacred Mountain Moisturizing Bar Soap, Sandalwood Moisture Cream, Satin Facial Scrub Mint, Sensation Bath & Shower Gel, Sensation Hand & Body Lotion, Sandalwood Moisture Cream, Sensation Massage Oil, Stevia Extract, Thieves Cleansing Bar Soap, Thieves Foaming Hand Soap, Thieves Waterless Hand Purifier, V-6 Enhanced Vegetable Oil Complex, Valor Moisturizing Bar Soap & Wolfberry Eye Cream. EOs: Acceptance, Bergamot, Dream Catcher, Egyptian Gold, Envision, Forgiveness, Frankincense, Galbanum, Gentle Baby, Geranium, Grapefruit, Gratitude, Helichrysum, Hope, Idaho tansy, Lavender, Lemon, Melaleuca, Melrose, Myrrh, Oregano, PaloSanto, Patchouli, Purification, Rose, Rosemary, Rosewood, Sacred Frankincense, Sandalwood, Western Red Cedar & Diffuser.

*(These statements have not been evaluated by the Food and Drug Administration. These products are not intended to diagnose, treat, cure or prevent any disease.)

Section 9

"It's not only children who grow. Parents do too. As much as we watch to see what our children do with their lives, they are watching us to see what we do with ours.

I can't tell my children to reach for the sun. All I can do is reach for it myself."

~ Joyce Maynard

YOUNG LIVING ESSENTIAL OILS

In your quest to promote your own long and healthy life, you will no doubt come across many good products produced by reputable companies. This has certainly been true for me, and I came to recognize that direct marketing companies usually build their reputations on the virtues of one or maybe a few flagship products of high quality. Young Living Essential Oils has built their reputation on quality not with just a few products, but over time with hundreds of products and a Distributorship devoted to sharing these products with others. Their flagship products are pure, unadulterated, Young Living Therapeutic-Grade™ (YLTG™) essential oils of which we may simply exclaim, "They work!"

Young Living has a mission statement and a company philosophy that motivates an ever growing number of essential oils- and health-conscious enthusiasts around the globe. They appreciate the quality standards maintained by Young Living and the unique business-building potential afforded to each member of the Young Living community. The direct marketing (also known as network marketing) structure fosters community as Distributors share the benefits of the products, the company and the pay plan with others.

Our legacy is to the children. The quote that introduces this Section was chosen as a way to express what happens in a home where YLTG™ essential oils are used. Children naturally gravitate to the oils. They are calmed and comforted by the combination of the pleasant fragrances and the touch of a loving hand applying the oils or offering nutritional supplements. This is an area of untold benefit that should not be underestimated when we count the blessings provided by this level of nurturing. Using the YLTG™ essential oils with our children whether by diffusing them in the living space or directly applying them, teaches children the gentle, more sensitive side to life in a world that is often less than sensitive to their needs. Of course, children of all ages appreciate these attributes, but the little ones are watching and learning from our examples and they remember.

Young Living does indeed have over 400 products from which to choose, and this is why I have listed them under body systems and uplifting emotions to give some indication of where you can begin to direct your personal research. When you are doing so, the question of how much you will have to invest to provide these helpful products will arise. This is a very personal and practical consideration. When looking to redirect some of your wellness budget to buy Young Living products, this statement by Unruh Publications may reinforce your desire toward your goals: "If you think that proper diet, food supplements, essential oils and herbs are too expensive - one way or another you will probably have to pay eventually anyway. It may be to the doctor or pharmacist. Even if this should happen, chances are that it will cost less in the long run. Our hope is that the life we save may be our own - and maybe someone else looking on!"[47]

We have experienced this very outcome in our lives. In the years before we began using the Young Living oral care products of *Thieves Dentarome Toothpaste* and *Thieves Fresh Essence Plus Mouthwash*, I had to take extra care with my gums and visit a dental hygienist every four months to avoid dental trouble. Not only was this extra expense, but there were several times when some form of intervention had to be performed that resulted in thousands of dollars in dental expenses. I have no idea of how much I have spent on *Thieves* products over the years, but I do know that I have not had one incident of gum problems in many years, and my regular schedule to visit the hygienist is now every six months with consistently healthy reports.

Dental health is also enjoyed by my husband, but his story involves an incident of very serious consequences that goes beyond the dollar amount spent over the years for oils like *Aroma Life* and supplements of *CardiaCare* and his daily *NingXia Red* juice. He carries a cardiovascular condition that has contributed to the early deaths of at least four close family members, and when he began experiencing chest pains we learned from the Cardiologist that one of his arteries that feeds the front of the heart was "hanging by a thread" yet he had not had a heart attack. The Cardiologist told us that knowing his history and because his body had developed a strong corollary artery that he "had already bought himself seven to ten years of life because of his lifestyle." Priceless!

We are so very grateful to Dr. Gary Young and his wife, Mary, for all they have done for us. This book would not have been written without their influence. They have encouraged each of us associated with Young Living to reach higher and to never give up. We don't know any others more dedicated to their goals or who work as hard as they do to achieve them.

ENHANCING WELLNESS WITH SCENT

Use of essential oils supports well being and contributes to inner harmony. Aromatherapy is a natural way to feel better using essential oils extracted from naturally aromatic plants. They help to bring balance to the whole being - spirit, mind and body.

For centuries, essential oils have been considered the most therapeutic and rejuvenating of all botanical extracts. Many recent scientific studies confirm the positive benefits of natural aromas reaching the brain directly through the olfactory nerve and limbic systems. It was my privilege when I was a Wellness Consultant to share clients' testimonies who had struggled with certain challenges, sometimes for years, until they found the key to unlock their emotions and gain release through fragrant applications of Young Living's therapeutic-grade essential oils.

YOUNG LIVING ESSENTIL OILS

Section 9: Table 1 - BENEFITS OF AROMATHERAPY

As highly concentrated distillates that carry oxygen, ozone and negative ions helping to create an environment where disease, bacteria, virus, etc., may not be able to live, 100% pure, therapeutic-quality essential oils are used for Aromatherapy as:

- anti-infectious, antiseptic, astringent...
- balancing, calming, digestive, disinfectant...
- elevating, energizing, euphoric, fortifying...
- invigorating, immuno-stimulant, to induce sleep...
- meditative, mental stimulant/clear thinking...
- memory, refreshing/purifying, rejuvenating...
- relaxing, revitalizing, tonic, regulating...
- stimulating, and warming.

BENEFITS OF YOUNG LIVING PRODUCTS

Concerning CMS and RWR, the various dynamics of my story must be told in the context of using Young Living products and the benefits my family and numerous friends have received, such as:

They have been immune enhancing.

They have supported our body's natural defenses.

They have been uplifting and mood elevating.

They have helped us receive spiritual insights.

They have strengthened our children and grandchildren.

Their high antioxidants have enhanced our health.

They have supported all of our body systems.

They have aided in maintaining cellular regeneration.

They have given us refreshing aromatic fragrance.

They have oxygenated and cleansed our air.

They have boosted our stamina and energy.

They have helped us relax and soothed sore muscles.

They have helped us manage stress and frustration.

They have helped the appearance of our skin and hair.

They have helped us improve mental clarity.

They have promoted overall vitality, and longevity.

They have helped us become slimmer.

They have helped us maintain healthy body weight.

They have attracted many new, like-minded friends.

They have blessed us with abundance in many ways.

THE PATH OF WELLNESS

My story appears to be ending, but it is truly a beginning too. What a pleasure it is to flow with each new day's adventures with energy and clarity of mind. It has taken me over three decades of stops and starts to arrive at this point, but I don't see it as if I have finished a journey. I've found a path to travel that suits me well.

You are invited to walk this path with me. We have an abundant selection of whole foods and Young Living products from which to choose to help us on our way. We can choose our words and watch over our hearts and thoughts. We can be aware of our bodies and the signals they send us. We can develop new, supportive habits, and we can be uplifted and inspired throughout the process as we cleanse and rebuild, cleanse and rebuild, cleanse and rebuild - enjoying life's adventure on our path of wellness.

When we think about the choices we have to make to stay on this path, there are times when we may not always be able to control the quality of the food that is available to us, but we can have control over the quality of essential oils and supplements we choose to put on and into our bodies. Isn't it a comforting thought to know that we can choose from Young Living's many quality products?

Another comforting thought about Young Living products is that they come with personal support of a Sponsor who will be dedicated to help you and encourage you on your path. Young Living Distributors are the friendliest, most sharing and giving group of people I have had the good fortune to meet and know. I began saying that sixteen years ago, and it holds true today.

If you are already a Member of the Young Living community of Customers and Distributors then you know what I mean about the people, and you are fortunate to have some knowledge and experience with the products and the company. You are aware of the many product choices available to you for each step of the CMS and RWR plans. It is my hope that you are inspired to walk the path too, and to take advantage of the superior formulations that Young Living has created to enhance wellness throughout the world.

If you are not a Member of Young Living, and would like to receive more information about the products or the company, contact the person who introduced you to this book. That person will be your Young Living Sponsor, if you wish, and he or she will help you get started. Besides your Sponsor and several upline Sponsors, there are company representatives dedicated to helping each Member and a Customer Care staff available too. Join us as we work and play to build a healthier world.

We are dedicated to follow-on with you and the Color Me Slim program so please visit our web site and blog and give us your comments and receive comments from others. May you be uplifted in heart and mind to believe you can achieve your very best state of wellness. Thank you, and I expect to be hearing from you. May you enjoy many fragrant blessings on your path to wellness!

YOUNG LIVING ESSENTIAL OILS
Section 9: Table 2 - ESSENTIAL OILS TO UPLIFT & INSPIRE

Speaking positive, uplifting, edifying words while breathing in the fragrances of the oils helps release stress and stored negative emotions. Choose two or three of the trigger words you identified when doing the first exercise in Section 1 (or any of the words you wish to choose to enhance positive energy), and note the italicized YLTG™ special blend that is known to help bring release and grounding

Wear these oils or diffuse them into your space. As you apply the particular oils, breathing in the fragrance, speak the word with intention to claim its full power.

Abundance (*Abundance*)
Adventure (*Live* with Passion)
Balance (*Valor* or *Grounding*)
Beauty (*Egyptian Gold*)
Believe (*Believe*)
Charity (*Sensation*)
Clarity (*Common Sense* or *Clarity*)
Communication (*Brain Power*)
Compassion (*Egyptian Gold*)
Consecration (*Humility*)
Courage (*Valor*)
Creativity (*Inspiration*)
Dedication (*3 Wise Men*)
Delight (*Present Time*)
Encourage (*Sacred Mountain*)
Endurance (*Motivation*)
Energy (**En-R-Gee**)
Enthusiasm (**Joy**)
Faith (*Envision*)
Flaithfulness (*Motivation*)
Favor (*White Angelica*)
Flexibility (*Acceptance*)
Forgiveness (*Forgiveness*)
Gladness (*Christmas Spirit*)

Gratitude (*Gratitude*)
Happiness (*Joy*)
Harmony (*Harmony*)
Health (*Legacy* or *Longevity*)
Healing (*Transformation*)
Honesty (*3 Wise Men*)
Hope (*Hope*)
Inspiration (*Inspiration*)
Integrity (*Legacy*)
Joy (*Joy*)
Patience (*Grounding*)
Peace (*Peace & Calming*)
Play (*Inner Child*)
Power (*Valor*)
Prosperity (*Abundance*)
Purpose (*Magnify Your Purpose*)
Release (*Release*)
Strength (*White Angelica*)
Tenderness (*Gentle Baby*)
Thanksgiving (*Gratitude*)
Truth (*Gathering*)
Understanding (*Awaken*)
Vision (*Awaken*)
Zest for Life (*Live with Passion*)

Section 10

"No matter where you are in life,
there is always more journey ahead."

~ Nelson Mandela

SUPPORT REFERENCES

Can you envision how Color Me Slim can be a viable plan for you? We are going to help by communicating with you through our blog. Join us as we share a wide range of ideas with free tips and strategies to help each other successfully meet our health goals. We welcome your comments and suggestions. Relating your experiences on the blog will give valuable inspiration to others. Please contribute often. The blog will be free to all, and will be monitored for accuracy and integrity.

From time-to-time we will announce further training or specialized support through webinar.

If you need help with placing an order or to receive notice of upcoming events, write us: info@ColorMeSlim.com

Subjects we intend to present are:

- A 90-Day Commitment to Your Health
- How to Save Money with Young Living Essential Rewards
- Sharing Color Me Slim with Others
- Business-Building and Color Me Slim
- Creating Abundance with the Young Living Commission and Bonus Plans
- The Young Living Share for Success System
- Earning Commissions while Reducing Weight and Getting Healthy

WEB REFERENCES

A simple Internet search will reveal a large selection for every health related subject that you can think of, as well as countless weight-reduction programs, tips, and recipes. Use these resources to your advantage to empower yourself.

For blog updates, support, and webinar schedules: www.ColorMeSlim.com

For Young Living Essential Oils: www.youngliving.com 800-371-2928

For literature and media pertinent to Young Living: www.ylwisdom.com and www.crowndiamondtools.com

Subscribe to receive e-news for discussions of up-to-date, natural source research by Dr. Al Sears, MD Dr. Sears also has a link to a current Glycemic Index: http://www.alsearsmd.com

Subscribe to Recipe-of-the-Day by Dr. Andrew Weil: www.drweil.com

Subscribe for discussions and blog of latest research on all matters of health and the environment by Dr. Joseph Mercola, DO: www.mercola.com

Subscribe to receive regular health and diet related emails. Very good, with titles such as: "7 Foods to Soothe Stress," "8 Ways to Eat More and Weigh Less" and "Fight Cravings Fast." Learn if you are biologically younger, older, or the same age as your calendar age: www.realage.com

For an excellent self-awareness test on the oxygen/stress connection and key oxygen information by O_2 The Oxygen Plan: www.theoxygenplan.com/stress

CMS & RWR

Section 10: Table 1 - TERMS TO RESEARCH

Artificial sweeteners:

Aspartame (Equal, NutraSweet, Canderel, and Amino Sweet).

Sucralose (Splenda).

Acesulfame K (Sunett, Sweet One).

Saccharin (Sweet 'N Low, Sugar Twin).

Fructose - especially high fructose corn syrup.

GMO - Educate yourself about Genetically Modified Organisms in our food supply and print a list of non-GMO companies and products to carry shopping: www.NonGMOShoppingGuide.com.

Hexane - solvent used to process soy products to render soy isolate and soy protein supplements.

MSG - For a resource about hidden sources of MSG find detailed listings at: www.msgmyth.com.

Pesticides - For information about natural pest control: www.beyondpesticides.com.

rBHT - hormones in our dairy foods.

Sulfates & sulfites - preservatives in prepared meats, deli, bacon, etc.

Toxins - For lists of toxic chemicals to avoid in food and the environment visit the Environmental Working Group site: http://ewg.org.

Triclosan - antibacterial agent in soap, also found in a wide variety of personal care and household products.

LITERATURE REFERENCES

Here is a partial list of author's works from which I have gleaned among them in their fields. You will find some that will be useful to you as you do your personal research.

✦ A Celebration of Vegetables - Menus for Festive Meat-Free Dining, by Robert Ackart

✦ Aromatherapy for the Soul - Spiritual and Emotional Empowerment with Essential Oils, by Judy Jehn, RMT

✦ Aromatherapy Scent and Psyche - Using Essential Oils for Physical and Emotional Well-Being, by Peter & Kate Damian

✦ Aromatherapy - The Essential Beginning, by D GaryYoung, ND

✦ Butterflies in a Bottle - How Essential Oils Free the Emotional Self and Liberate the Body/Mind, by Gregory T. Hitter, PhD

✦ Changing for Good - A Revolutionary Six-Stage Program for Overcoming Bad Habits and Moving Your Life Positively Forward, by James Prochaska, PhD, John Norcross, PhD, Carlo Diclemente, PhD

✦ Different Bodies Different Diets - Losing Weight Is as Easy as Finding Your Body Type, by Carolyn Mein, D C

✦ Discovery of the Ultimate Superfood - How the NingXia Wolfberry and Four Other Whole Foods Help Combat Heart Disease, Cancer, Chronic Fatigue, Depression, Diabetes and More, by Gary Young, ND, Ronald Lawrence, MD, PhD and Marc Schreuder

✦ Dr. DeMarco Answers Your Questions, by Dr. Carolyn DeMarco, MD

- Energetics of Food - Encounters with Your Most Intimate Relationship, by Steve Gagne'

- Essential Oils Desk Reference, compiled by Essential Science Publishing, Distributed by Y L Wisdom

- Feelings Buried Alive Never Die, by Karol K. Truman

- Food Enzymes for Vibrant Health and Increased Longevity - Rejuvenate, Reinvigorate, and Revitalize Your Body with the Gift of Enzymes, by Tonita d'Raye

- Food Healing for Man, by Bernard Jensen, PhD

- Foods That Make You Lose Weight - Or Negative Calories, by Isabelle Martin

- Harmony, Joy & Abundance - Mastering the Art and the Language of Sharing Young Living Essential Oils, by Vicki H. Opfer

- Healing Feelings from Your Heart, by Karol K. Truman

- Healing Oils Healing Hands - Discovering the Power of Prayer, Hands on Healing and Anointing, by Linda L. Smith, RN

- Healing Oils of the Bible, by David Stewart, PhD

- Holistic Aromatherapy for Animals - A Comprehensive Guide to the Use of Essential Oils & Hydrosols with Animals, by Kristen Leigh Bell

- In Fitness and in Health - Everyone Is an Athlete, by Dr. Philip Maffetone, DC

- Inner Transformations Using Essential Oils - Powerful Cleansing Protocols for Increased Energy and Better Health, by Dr. LeAnne Deardeuff, DC & Dr. David Deardeuff, DC

+ Integrating Your Wholeness - A Reference Guide to Assist You in Merging with Your Internal Physician, by Rev. Marcy Foley, DC, ND

+ Listening and Communicating with Energy - Understanding Energies and Your Own Intuitive Nature, by Ginger Bowler, PhD

+ Live Better Longer - The Parcells Center 7-Step Plan for Health and Longevity, by Joseph Dispenza

+ Magnificent Mind at Any Age - Treat Anxiety, Depression, Memory Problems, ADD, and Insomnia, by Dr. Daniel G. Amen, MD

+ Molecules of Emotion - The Science Behind Mind-Body Medicine, by Dr. Candace B. Pert, MD

+ Real Fibromyalgia Rx -Targeting the Pituitary as the Root Cause, by Dr. Dan Purser, MD

+ Real Food - What to Eat and Why, by Nina Planck

+ Real Solutions for the Top 7 Female Health Concerns, by Dr. Dan Purser, MD

+ Rebounding to Better Health - A Practical Guide to the Ultimate Exercise, by Linda Brooks, CR

+ Releasing Emotional Patterns with Essential Oils, by Carolyn L. Mein, DC

+ Saving Face - The Scents-Able Way to Wrinkle-Free Skin, by Dr. Sabina DeVita

+ Scriptural Essence - Temple Secrets Revealed, by Janet McBride

+ Take Charge of Your Body, by Dr. Carolyn DeMarco, MD

+ Take Control of Your Health - Your Proven Guide to Peak Wellness and Ideal Weight, by Dr. Joseph Mercola, DO

+ The Acid Alkaline Balance Diet - An Innovative Program for Ridding Your Body of Acidic Wastes, by Felicia Drury Kliment

+ The Chemistry of Man, by Bernard Jensen, PhD

+ The China Study - Startling Implications for Diet, Weight Loss and Long-Term Health, by T. Colin Campbell, PhD and Thomas M. Campbell, II

+ The Coconut Oil Miracle, by Bruce Fife, CN, ND

+ The Cortisol Connection - Why Stress Makes You Fat and Ruins Your Health and What You Can Do About It, by Shawn Talbott, Ph.D.

+ The pH Miracle for Weight Loss - Balance Your Body Chemistry, Achieve Your Ideal Weight, by Robert O. Young, PhD and Shelley Redford Young

+ The No-Grain Diet - Conquer Carbohydrate Addiction & Stay Slim for Life, by Dr. Joseph Mercola, DO

+ The Raw 50, by Carol Alt

+ The Raw Food Feast - 7 Days Through the Rainbow, by Mandilyn Canistelle

+ The Step Diet Book - Count Steps, Not Calories, to Lose Weight and Keep It Off Forever, by James O. Hill, PhD and John C. Peters, PhD

+ Why Do I Still Have Thyroid Symptoms When My Lab Tests Are Normal?, by Datis Kharranzian, DHSc, DC, MS

+ Your Body's Many Cries for Water - You Are Not Sick, You Are Thirsty! by F. Batmanghelidj, MD

INDEX OF TABLES BY SECTION

BIBLIOGRAPHY

[1] Mein, Carolyn, D.C., <u>Releasing Emotional Patterns with Essential oils</u>, Vision Ware Press, Rancho Santa Fe, CA. July, 1998. p 3.

[2] Walke, Hilary, "Oprah's Epiphany: 'I'm Never Dieting Again.'" That's Fit, Diet & Weight Loss Celebs & Entertainment May 10, 2010.

[3] Damian, Peter & Kate, <u>Aromatherapy Scent and Psyche-Using Essential Oil for Physical and Emotional Well Being</u>, Healing Arts Press, Rochester, VT. 1995. pgs 74-76.

[4] "Weight Control and Diet," Health Topics A-Z www.about.com, http://adam.about.com/reports/

[5] Barnes P. M., Bloom B., Nahin R. CDC National Health Statistics, #12. Nov 19, 2009.

[6] http://www.disabled-world.com/medical/alternative/holistic/care-statistics.php

[7] Gagne, Steve, <u>Energetics of Food - Encounters with Your Most Intimate Relationship</u>, Spiral Sciences, Santa Fe, NM. 1990. p 11.

[8] http://www.cdc.gov/nchs/products/pubs/pubd/hestats/obese/obse99.htm and http://www.obesity.org/statistics/

[9] http://www.bioscience.org/news/scientis/obesity2.htm

[10] www.about.com: Health Topics A-Z, Weight Control and Diet. http://adam.about.com/reports/000053_3.htm

[11] http://www.fruitsandveggiesmatter.gov/

[12] Jensen, Bernard, <u>Food Healing for Man</u>, "Foods and Color Healing." Bernard Jensen Publisher, Escondido, CA, 1983. pgs 69-71.

[13] Gagne', Steve, <u>Energetics of Food - Encounters with Your Most Intimate Relationship</u>, Spiral Sciences, Santa Fe, NM. 1990. p 42.

[13] http://www.cdc.gov/nchs/products/pubs/pubd/hestats/obese/obse99.htm

[14] www.cdc.gov/nccdphp/dnpa/nutrition/pdf/portion_size_research.pdf

[15] http://www.health.gov/dietaryguidelines/dga2005/document/html/appendixA.htm#foota

[16] The Traffic Light Diet, www.adaevidencelibrary.com/topic.cfm?cat=1429

[17] http://articles.mercola.com/sites/articles/archive/2010/04/20/sugar-dangers.aspx

[18] Jensen, Bernard, <u>Tissue Cleansing Through Bowel Management</u>, Bernard Jensen International, Escondido, CA. 1981.

[19] Getting Rid of the Toxins in Your Home and Your Body, "Body Burden, the Pollution in People," Environmental Working Group," 2002. See http://archive.ewg.org/reports/bodyburden1/es.php.

[20] Jensen, Bernard, <u>Tissue Cleansing Through Bowel Management</u>, Bernard Jensen International, Escondido, CA. 1981.

[21] Getting Rid of the Toxins in Your Home and Your Body, "Body Burden, the Pollution in People," Environmental Working Group," 2002. See http://archive.ewg.org/reports/bodyburden1/es.php

[22] Bass, Stanley S., N.D., D.C., Ph.C., "What Symptoms to Expect When You Improve Your Diet." Seminar handout. p 7.

[23] www.dictionary.com

[24] http://www.nlm.nih.gov/medlineplus/stress.html

[25] http://www.apa.org/helpcenter/stress-signs.aspx

[26] Ibid.

[27] www.nlm.nih.gov/medlineplus/news/
fullstory_97459.html

[28] Ibid.

[29] The Holy Bible, Ephesians 4:26.

[30] Mercola, Joseph. "The Major Exercise Mistake I Made for Over 30 Years..." http://fitness.mercola.com/sites/fitness/archive/2010/06/26/10-minutes-of-exercise-yields-hourlong-effects.aspx. June 26, 2010

[31] Ibid.

[32] Mercola, Joseph. http://articles.mercola.com/sites/articles/archive/2010/04/13/should-you-eat-many-small-meals-each-day.aspx April 13, 2010.

[33] Jensen, Bernard, Food Healing for Man, "Does the Physical Body Possess Life." Bernard Jensen Publisher, Escondido, CA. 1983. p 65.

[34] The Holy Bible, Leviticus 17:11

[35] Batmanghelidj, F., M.D., Your Body's Many Cries for Water, Global Health Solutions, Inc., Falls Church, VA. Feb, 1997. p 99.

[36] Ibid. p 3-4.

[37] The Holy Bible, Leviticus 17:11.

[38] Mercola, Joseph, The No-Grain Diet-Conquer Carbohydrate Addiction and Stay Slim for Life, Penguin Books, NY, NY. April, 2004. p 119.

[39] Ibid, p 119.

[40] "FDA Should Set Standards for Salt Added to Processed Foods, Prepared Meals," National Academy of Sciences, Office of News and Public Information. April 20, 2010. www.nasonline.org/site/PageServer?JServSessionIdr004...1

[41] "A sweet problem: Princeton researchers find that high-fructose corn syrup prompts considerably more weight gain. News at Princeton. March 22, 2010. http://www.princeton.edu/main/news/archive/S26/91/22K07/index.xml?section=newsreleases

[42] Ibid.

[43] Ibid. "Reduce Sugar, Improve Cholesterol," May 4, 2010. http://www.newsmaxhealth.com/vera_tweed/reduce_sugar_cholesterol/2010/05/04/315009.html

[44] Mercola, Joseph. "Which Veggie Burgers Were Made with a Neurotoxin?"www.Mercola.com. May 15, 2010.

[45] Canistelle, Mandilyn. The Raw Food Feast - 7 Days Through the Rainbow, Growing Healthy Homes, LLC, Bartlesville, OK. 2010. pgs 27-29.

[46] Adapted from School Handout, untitled, author unknown.

[47] "Health Is Learned-Health Is Earned," Unruh Publication, Sioux Falls, SD. Seminar Handout.